Encyclopedia of Oral and Maxillofacial Surgery

Volume II

Encyclopedia of Oral and Maxillofacial Surgery Volume II

Edited by **Dave Clark**

FOSTER
A C A D E M I C S

New Jersey

Published by Foster Academics,
61 Van Reypen Street,
Jersey City, NJ 07306, USA
www.fosteracademics.com

Encyclopedia of Oral and Maxillofacial Surgery
Volume II
Edited by Dave Clark

International Standard Book Number: 978-1-63242-002-2 (Hardback)

Printed in the United States of America.

Contents

Preface   VII

Section 1   Maxillofacial Fractures: Diagnosis and Management   1

Chapter 1   **Management of Midfacial Fractures**   3
             Sertac Aktop, Onur Gonul, Tulin Satilmis, Hasan Garip and
             Kamil Goker

Chapter 2   **Management of Mandibular Fractures**   34
             Amrish Bhagol, Virendra Singh and Ruchi Singhal

Section 2   **Advanced Maxillofacial Distraction Osteogenesis:**
             State-of-the-Art   64

Chapter 3   **Distraction Osteogenesis**   66
             Hossein Behnia, Azita Tehranchi and Golnaz Morad

Section 3   Advanced Oral and Maxillofacial Reconstruction   96

Chapter 4   **Microsurgical Reconstruction of Maxillary Defects**   98
             Shahram Nazerani

Chapter 5   **Reconstruction of Mandibular Defects**   128
             Maiolino Thomaz Fonseca Oliveira, Flaviana Soares Rocha, Jonas
             Dantas Batista, Sylvio Luiz Costa de Moraes and Darceny Zanetta-
             Barbosa

Chapter 6   **Maxillofacial Reconstruction of Ballistic Injuries**   148
             Mohammad Hosein Kalantar Motamedi, Seyed Hossein Mortazavi,
             Hossein Behnia, Masoud Yaghmaei, Abbas Khodayari, Fahimeh
             Akhlaghi, Mohammad Ghasem Shams and Rashid Zargar Marandi

Chapter 7   **Cleft Lip and Palate Surgery**   175
             Koroush Taheri Talesh and Mohammad Hosein Kalantar Motamedi

Chapter 8   **Current Advances in Mandibular Condyle**
             Reconstruction   189
             Tarek El-Bialy and Adel Alhadlaq

Chapter 9   **The Cosmetic Considerations in Facial Defect**
             Reconstruction   210
             Mazen Almasri

             Permissions

             List of Contributors

Preface

This book has been a concerted effort by a group of academicians, researchers and scientists, who have contributed their research works for the realization of the book. This book has materialized in the wake of emerging advancements and innovations in this field. Therefore, the need of the hour was to compile all the required researches and disseminate the knowledge to a broad spectrum of people comprising of students, researchers and specialists of the field.

The discipline of oral and maxillofacial surgery includes a broad range of diseases, conditions, injuries and deformities of the head, neck, face and jaws along with the hard and soft tissues of the oral cavity. It is an internationally acknowledged surgical attribute rapidly growing with new developments in technology. New handbooks are required to keep practitioners updated of the developments made world-wide. This book aims to present progressive researches on complex issues examined under the following sections namely, Maxillofacial Fractures: Diagnosis and Management, Advanced Maxillofacial Distraction Osteogenesis, and Advanced Oral and Maxillofacial Reconstruction.

At the end of the preface, I would like to thank the authors for their brilliant chapters and the publisher for guiding us all-through the making of the book till its final stage. Also, I would like to thank my family for providing the support and encouragement throughout my academic career and research projects.

Editor

Maxillofacial Fractures: Diagnosis and Management

Management of Midfacial Fractures

Sertac Aktop, Onur Gonul, Tulin Satilmis,
Hasan Garip and Kamil Goker

Additional information is available at the end of the chapter

1. Introduction

The management of midfacial fractures includes the treatment of facial fractures, dentoalveolar trauma, and soft-tissue injuries, as well as associated injuries, mainly of the head and neck [1]. The management of fractures of the maxillofacial complex remains a challenge for the oral maxillofacial surgeon, demanding both skill and expertise [2]. The success of treatment and implementation of preventive measures are more specifically dependent on epidemiologic assessments [3].Midfacial fractures can occur in isolation or in combination with other serious injuries, including mandibular, ophthalmologic, cranial, spinal, thoracic, and abdominal trauma, as well as upper and lower orthopedic injuries [4].The epidemiology of facial fractures varies in type, severity, and cause depending on the population studied. Differences among populations in the causes of maxillofacial fractures may be the result of differences in risk and cultural factors among countries, but are more likely to be influenced by the severity of injury [1,5]. The causes of maxillofacial fractures have changed over the past three decades, and they continue to do so. The main causes worldwide are traffic accidents, assaults, falls, sport-related injuries, and warfare [6-8]. Many articles pertaining to the incidence and causes of maxillofacial injuries have been published [1,4,7-10]. In 2003, Motamedi [7] reported the distribution of facial fractures as 72.9% mandibular, 13.9% maxillary, 13.5% zygomatic, 24.0% zygomatico-orbital, 2.1% cranial, 2.1% nasal, and 1.6% frontal injuries [Figure 1].

Causes of these maxillofacial injuries were automobile (30.8%) and motorcycle (23.2%) accidents, altercations (9.7%), sport (6.3%), and warfare (9.7%) [Figure 2].

The distribution of maxillary fractures was 54.6% Le Fort II, 24.2% Le Fort I, 12.1% Le Fort III, and 9.1% alveolar [7] [Figure 3].

According to Cook and Rowe [4], midfacial injuries occur most frequently in individuals aged 21–30 years (43%). The 11–20-year and 31–40-year age groups each account for 20% of these

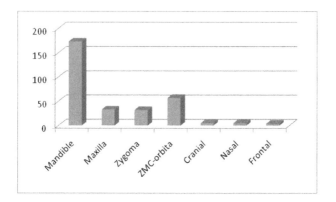

Figure 1. Fracture sites are shown for 237 maxillofacial trauma patients according to Motamedi

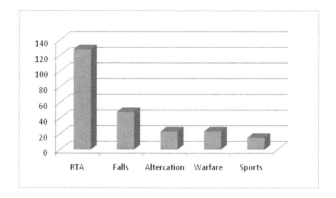

Figure 2. The causes of fracture for Motamedi's assessment of maxillofacial trauma patients

fractures. Most (83.1%) midfacial fractures occur in males, with the remainder (16.9%) occurring in females [4] [Figure 4].

Thoren [9] noted that injuries are associated with 25.2% of midfacial fractures. These injuries most commonly affect a limb (13.5%), followed by the brain (11.0%), chest (5.5%), spine (2.7%), and abdomen (0.8%) [9].

2. Surgical anatomy

The anatomy of the head is complex; the physical properties of the skin, bone, and brain differ markedly and the facial skeletal components articulate and interdigitate in a complex fashion, with the consequence that a given facial bone is rarely fractured without disrupting its

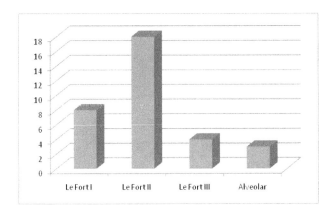

Figure 3. Distribution of maxillary fractures in Motamedi's assessment of maxillofacial trauma patients

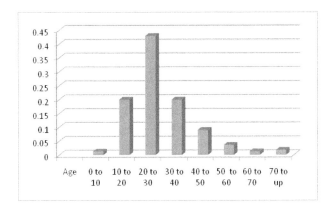

Figure 4. Age distribution of midfacial fracture patients according to Cook and Rowe.

neighbor [10]. The severity and pattern of a fracture depend on the magnitude of the causative force, impact duration, the acceleration imparted by impact to the affected part of the body, and the rate of acceleration change. The surface area of the impact site is also relevant [11,12]. The middle third of the facial skeleton is defined as an area bounded superiorly by a line drawn across the skull from the zygomaticofrontal suture, across the frontonasal and frontomaxillary sutures, to the zygomaticofrontal suture on the opposite side; and inferiorly by the occlusal plane of the maxillary teeth, or, in an edentulous patient, by the maxillary alveolar ridge. It extends posteriorly to the frontal bone in the superior region and the body of the sphenoid in the inferior region, and the pterygoid plates of the sphenoid are usually involved in any severe fracture [13].

The middle third of the facial skeleton comprises the following bones [14] [Figure 5]:

- Two maxillae
- Two zygomatic bones
- Two zygomatic processes of the temporal bones
- Two palatine bones
- Two nasal bones
- Two lacrimal bones
- The vomer
- The ethmoid and attached conchae
- Two inferior conchae
- The pterygoid plates of the sphenoid

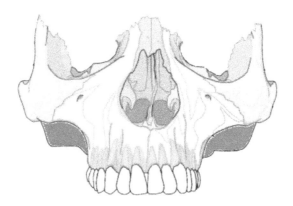

Figure 5. Bones of the middle third of the facial skeleton

The frontal bone and the sphenoid body and greater and lesser wings are not usually fractured. In fact, they are protected to a considerable extent by the cushioning effect achieved as the fracturing force crushes the comparatively weak bones comprising the middle third of the facial skeleton [13].

3. Initial management of the midfacial trauma patient

The initial assessment and management of a patient's injuries must be completed in an accurate and systematic manner to quickly establish the extent of any damage to vital life-support systems. Patients are assessed and treatment priorities are established based on patients' injuries and the stability of their vital signs. Injuries can be divided into three general categories: severe, urgent, and non-urgent. Severe injuries are immediately life threatening and interfere with vital physiologic functions; examples are compromised airway, inadequate breathing, hemorrhage, and circulatory system damage or shock. These injuries constitute approximately 5% of patient injuries but represent more than 50% of injuries associated with all trauma deaths. Urgent injuries make up approximately 10–15% of all injuries and present no immediate threat to life. Patients with this type of injury may present with damage to the abdomen, orofacial structures, chest, or extremities that requires surgical intervention or repair, but their vital signs are stable. Non-urgent injuries account for approximately 80% of all injuries and are not immediately life threatening. Patients with this type of trauma eventually require surgical or medical management, although the exact nature of the injury may not become apparent until significant evaluation and observation are performed. The goal of initial emergency care is to provide life-saving and support measures until definitive care can be initiated. Any trauma victim with altered consciousness must be considered to have a brain injury. The level of consciousness is assessed by serial Glasgow Coma Scale evaluations [15] [Table 1].

Action	Score
Eye Opening	4
Spontaneous	3
To speech	2
To pain	1
None	6
Motor Response	5
Obeys	4
Localises pain	3
Withdraws from pain	2
Flexion to pain	1
Extension to pain	5
None	4
Verbal Response	3
Oriented	2
Confused	1
Inappropriate	
Incomprehensible	
None	

Adapted from Teasdale and Jennett [15]. A patient's score determines the category of neurologic impairment: 15 = normal, 13 or 14 = mild injury, 9–12 = moderate injury, and 3–8 = severe injury.

Table 1. Glasgow Coma Scale.

Other signs of brain damage include restlessness, convulsions, and cranial nerve dysfunction (*e.g.* a nonreactive pupil). The classic Cushing triad (hypertension, bradycardia, and respiratory disturbances) is a late and unreliable sign that usually closely precedes brain herniation. Hypotension is rarely due to head injury alone. Patients suspected of sustaining head trauma should not receive any premedication that will alter their mental status (*e.g.* sedatives or analgesics) or neurologic examination (*e.g.* anticholinergic-induced pupillary dilation).

3.1. Primary Survey: ABCs

During the primary survey, life-threatening conditions are identified and reversed quickly. This period calls for quick and efficient evaluation of the patient's injuries and almost simultaneous life-saving intervention. The primary survey progresses in a logical manner based on the ABC pneumonic: airway maintenance with cervical spine control, breathing and adequate ventilation, and circulation with control of hemorrhage. The letters D and E have also been added: a brief neurologic examination to establish the degree of consciousness, and exposure of the patient *via* complete undressing to avoid overlooking injuries camouflaged by clothing. Maxillofacial injuries may result in airway compromise caused by any of several factors: blood and secretions, a mandibular fracture that allows the tongue to fall against the posterior wall of the pharynx, a midfacial injury that causes the maxilla to fall posteroinferiorly into the nasopharynx, and foreign debris such as avulsed teeth or dentures. A large tonsillar suction tip should be used to clear the oral cavity and pharynx. The establishment of an oral airway assists with tongue position; however, care must always be taken to avoid manipulation of the neck and to provide access to the oral cavity and dentition for the reduction and fixation of any fractures requiring a period of intermaxillary fixation. Neither midfacial fractures nor cerebrospinal rhinorrhea are contraindications to nasal intubation. Care should be taken to pass the tube along the nasal floor into the pharynx, and the tube should be visualised before tracheal intubation. Hypertension or tachycardia during intubation can be attenuated with the intravenous administration of lidocaine or fentanyl. Intubation while the patient is awake causes a precipitous rise in intracranial pressure. Nasal passage of an endotracheal or nasogastric tube in a patient with a basal skull fracture risks cribriform plate perforation and cerebrospinal fluid infection. Slight elevation of the head will improve venous drainage and decrease intracranial pressure.

3.2. Physical examination

The physical examination should begin with an evaluation of soft-tissue injuries. Lacerations should be debrided and examined for disruption of vital structures, such as the facial nerve or parotid duct. The eyelids should be elevated to allow evaluation of the eyes for neurologic and ocular damage. The face should be symmetric, without discolouration or swelling suggestive of bony or soft-tissue injury. The bony landmarks should be palpated, beginning with the supraorbital and lateral orbital rims and followed by the infraorbital rims, malar eminences, zygomatic arches, and nasal bones. Any steps or irregularities along the bony margin are suggestive of a fracture. Numbness over the area of distribution of the trigeminal nerve is usually noted with fractures of the facial skeleton. The oral cavity should be inspected and evaluated for lost teeth, lacerations, and occlusal alterations. Any tooth lost at the time of injury must be accounted for because it may have been aspirated or swallowed. The neck should also be examined for injury. Subcutaneous air may be visualised if massive injury is present; if subtle, it may be detected only by palpation. The presence of air in the soft tissue may be the result of tracheal damage. Any externally expanding edema or hematoma of the neck must be observed closely for continued expansion and airway compromise. Carotid pulses should be assessed. Palpation should be performed to detect abnormalities in the contour of the thyroid cartilage and to confirm the midline position of the trachea in the suprasternal notch.

3.3. Preoperative considerations

Patients with midfacial trauma often pose the greatest airway challenges to the anaesthesiologist. Preoperative airway evaluation must be detailed and thorough. Particular attention should be focused on jaw opening, mask fit, neck mobility, maxillary protrusion, macroglossia, dental pathology, nasal patency, and the existence of any intraoral lesion or debris. If any forewarning sign of problems with mask ventilation or endotracheal intubation is observed, the airway should be secured prior to anaesthesia induction. This process may involve fibreoptic nasal or oral intubation or tracheostomy. Nasal intubation with a preformed or straight tube with a flexible angle connector is usually preferred in dental or oral surgery. The endotracheal tube can then be directed cephalically and connected to breathing tubes passing over the patient's head.

3.4. Intraoperative management

Reconstructive surgery can be associated with substantial blood loss. Strategies to minimise bleeding include a slight head-up position, controlled hypotension, and local infiltration with epinephrine solutions. Because the patient's arms are typically tucked along the sides of the body, at least two intravenous lines should be established prior to surgery. This step is especially important if one line is used for the delivery of an anaesthetic or hypotensive agent. An arterial line can be helpful in cases of marked blood loss, as a surgeon leaning against the patient's arm may interfere with non-invasive blood pressure cuff readings. An oropharyngeal pack is often placed to minimize the amount of blood and other debris reaching the larynx and trachea. Due to the proximity of the airway to the surgical field, the anaesthesiologist's location is more remote than usual. This situation increases the likelihood of serious intraoperative airway problems, such as endotracheal tube kinking, disconnection, or perforation by a surgical instrument. Airway monitoring of end-tidal CO_2, peak inspiratory pressures, and esophageal stethoscope breath sounds assumes increased importance in such cases. At the end of the surgery, the oropharyngeal pack must be removed and the pharynx suctioned. Although the presence of some bloody debris during initial suctioning is not unusual, repeated efforts should be less productive. If there is a chance of postoperative edema involving structures that could potentially obstruct the airway (e.g. the tongue), the patient should be left intubated. Otherwise, extubation can be attempted once the patient is fully awake and shows no sign of continued bleeding. Appropriate cutting tools should be placed at the bedside of a patient with intermaxillary fixation (*e.g.* maxillomandibular wiring), in case of vomiting or other airway emergency.

4. Dentoalveolar fractures

Fracture of the alveolar process is a common injury, comprising 2–8% of all craniofacial injuries. Nearby soft tissues and teeth are often damaged, increasing the severity of the situation [16]. The most common causes of such fractures are falls, motor vehicle accidents, sporting injuries, altercations, child abuse, and playground accidents. Direct or indirect force on a tooth, the latter transmitted most commonly through overlying soft tissues, may cause dentoalveolar injury [17].

4.1. Clinical examination

The practitioner should first ask when, where, and how the injury occurred and whether any treatment has been provided since that time. Answers to these simple questions could provide important clues. The patient's general health status should be known and his or her current situation examined when any nausea, vomiting, unconsciousness, amnesia, headache, or visual disturbance has occurred after injury. The examination of a patient's dentoalveolar injuries should assess the condition of the extraoral and intraoral soft tissues, jaws, and alveolar bone; establish the presence of any tooth displacement or mobility; and include tooth percussion and pulp testing [18]. Lacerations, abrasions, and contusions are very common in dentoalveolar injuries. Any vital structure crossing the line of laceration should be noted. The removal of blood clots, saline irrigation, and cleaning of the oral cavity facilitate inspection. Any foreign body within surrounding tissues should be examined carefully because bone or tooth fragments might have penetrated these areas, depending on the mechanism of injury. All fractured or missing teeth and restorations should be assumed to have been swallowed, aspirated, or lodged in adjacent structures. Alveolar segment fractures can be detected readily by visual examination and palpation. However, examination may be difficult because of post-injury pain. Sublingual ecchymosis on the mouth floor is pathognomonic for an underlying mandibular fracture. Step defects, crepitation, malocclusion, and gingival lacerations should raise the suspicion of possible underlying bony defects. The presence of fractured teeth should be noted. The depth of the fracture is very important. Complete mobility of the crown may indicate crown–root fracture. Post-injury occlusion should be checked and any displacement, intrusion, or luxation should be examined carefully. Percussion tests to determine sensitivity and pulp vitality should be performed to rule out periodontal ligament injury and many types of tooth fracture.

4.2. Imaging

Radiographic studies should be performed before intraoral manipulation. Radiography should determine the presence of root or jaw fracture, degree of extrusion or intrusion and its relationship to possible existing tooth germs, extent of root development, and presence of tooth fragments and foreign bodies lodged in soft tissues. The combination of periapical, occlusal, and panoramic radiographs is used most frequently for the detection of damage to underlying tissues. Periapical radiographs provide the most detailed information about root fractures and tooth dislocation. Occlusal radiographs, however, provide larger fields of view and nearly the same level of detail as periapical radiographs; they are also very useful for the detection of foreign bodies. Panoramic radiographs provide useful screening views and visualize fractures of the mandible, maxilla, alveolar ridges, and teeth. Computed tomography (CT) offers insufficient resolution for the diagnosis of dental trauma, but cone-beam CT technology provides sufficient resolution to serve as a valuable tool in the diagnosis of various dental injuries [17,19,20].

4.3. Classification

The most commonly used simple and comprehensive classification of dentoalveolar injuries was developed by Andreasen [21] [Figure 6].

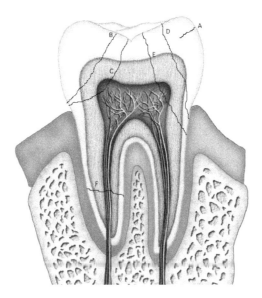

Figure 6. Diagram of Andreasen's classification

Dental tissues and pulp

- Simple crown infraction (crack in the tooth without loss of tooth substance)
- Uncomplicated crown fracture (confined to enamel, or enamel and dentine, with no root exposure)
- Complicated crown fracture (pulp exposure)

- Uncomplicated crown–root fracture (involving the enamel, dentine, and cementum without pulp exposure)

- Complicated crown–root fracture (involving the enamel, dentine, and cementum with pulp exposure)

- Root fracture (involving the dentine and cementum with pulp exposure)

Injuries to periodontal tissues

- Concussion: injury to the periodontium producing sensitivity to percussion without tooth loosening or displacement

- Subluxation: the tooth is loosened but not displaced

- Extrusive luxation, lateral luxation, intrusive luxation

- Avulsion: tooth displacement without accompanying comminution or fracture of the alveolar socket

Injuries to the supporting bone

- Comminution of the alveolar housing, often with intrusive or lateral luxation

- Fracture of a single wall of an alveolus

- Fracture of the alveolar process *en bloc* in a dentate patient; the fracture line does not necessarily extend through a tooth socket

- Fracture involving the main body of the mandible or maxilla

4.4. Treatment

The aim of dentoalveolar fracture treatment is to re-establish the normal form and function of the masticatory system. The involvement of pulp tissue makes a great difference in the treatment protocol.

4.4.1. Dental tissues and pulp

Simple crown infractions do not require treatment. Multiple cracks can be sealed with restorative materials to prevent staining. For uncomplicated crown fractures affecting only the enamel, grinding of the sharp edges is one possible solution. In cases of extensive enamel loss, a composite restoration may be used for recontouring. If a considerable amount of dentine is exposed, it should be covered with glass ionomer as an emergency treatment, and permanent composite restoration with bonding agents can be performed immediately or at a later stage. If the missing fragment is found, bonding to the tooth can be attempted with dentine bonding agents. Periodic follow-up visits should be scheduled to monitor pulp vitality. The management of complicated crown fractures is more challenging. If the exposed pulp tissue is vital, pulp capping or pulpotomy should be performed in cases without extensive crown loss. In cases of severe loss of crown substance or a lengthy interval between injury and treatment, pulp extirpation should be performed *via* $Ca(OH)_2$ application in the root canal. Permanent root canal filling is carried out later in such cases. If the exposed pulp tissue is already necrotic, $Ca(OH)_2$ should be applied immediately after canal debridement. The course of treatment for uncomplicated crown–root fractures depends on the fracture location. An intact coronal fragment must be removed and inspected carefully to determine whether restoration of the remaining fragment is possible. If the fracture does not extend too far apically, the remaining fragment is suitable for restoration, and the pulp has not been exposed, the treatment protocol is the same as described above for crown fractures. Gingivectomy, ostectomy, or orthodontic extrusion might be required later for tooth restoration. In complicated crown–root fractures, pulp extirpation and $Ca(OH)_2$ application are recommended during the emergency stage, followed by the permanent restoration of the remaining tooth fragment after root canal filling. Surgical extrusion is an option for such fractures because the pulp tissue cannot be devitalised as in uncomplicated crown–root fractures. When no combination of procedures successfully renders the remaining fragment restorable, extraction of the tooth is necessary. When root fractures are located above or close to the gingival crevice, the whole tooth should be extracted; when the remaining tissue allows tooth restoration, only the coronal fragment should be removed for root canal therapy and post and core restoration. Fractures between the middle and apical thirds of the tooth have a good prognosis for pulp survival and the joining of root fragments to one another during healing. A displaced or mobile fragment should be repositioned correctly and the tooth should be splinted for 2–3 months. During this time, the fragments usually calcify. The tooth should be inspected for signs of pulp necrosis during follow-up visits and root canal therapy should be performed if necessary.

4.4.2. Injuries to periodontal tissues

Concussed teeth present only tenderness to percussion in the horizontal and vertical directions. Removing the tooth from occlusion is the only accepted treatment option in such cases. Subluxated teeth show no clinical or radiographic displacement, but damage to the periodontal ligament tissue is present. Periodontal tissue rupture can cause bleeding from the gingival margin crevice. Treatment in these cases is the same as described for concussion, and follow-up monitoring of pulp vitality is necessary. Extrusive luxation is characterized by neurovascular and periodontal ligament rupture with mobility and bleeding from the gingival margin. Pulp necrosis and external root resorption may be seen in later stages. The tooth should be positioned properly and splinted to uninjured adjacent teeth with an acid-etch/resin splint for 3 weeks. Other methods of splinting used routinely in oral and maxillofacial surgery are not recommended. If pulp necrosis occurs, endodontic therapy should be performed. Lateral extrusions often involve the alveolar bone, and may be characterized by complex gingival lacerations and step deformities. The goal of treatment is to properly reposition the alveolar bone and tooth, which can be accomplished with the application of an acid-etch/resin splint for 4–8 weeks. Intrusive luxation is characterized by obvious tooth displacement and comminution and fracture of the alveolus. The risks of pulpal necrosis and inflammatory root resorption are higher in such cases than in other dentoalveolar injuries. Affected teeth with complete root development and closed apices should be repositioned and stabilized with a non-rigid splint. Endodontic therapy within 10–14 days after injury, including canal filling with $Ca(OH)_2$, is recommended to retard or inhibit the inflammatory or replacement resorption process. Intrusion of an incompletely developed tooth is discussed in the 'Midfacial Fractures in Children' section below. The fate of an avulsed tooth depends on the cellular viability of the periodontal fibres that remain attached to the root surface prior to reimplantation. Important factors determining the success of treatment measures are the length of time that the tooth has been out of the socket, the state of the tooth and periodontal tissues, and the manner in which the tooth has been preserved before replantation. Avulsed teeth should be stored temporarily in milk, saliva, saline, or Hank's solution. More than 15 min of extraoral exposure of a periodontal ligament will deplete most cell metabolites in the dental tissue. Teeth in poor hygienic condition and those with moderate to severe periodontal disease, gross caries involving the pulp, apical abscess, infection at the replanting site, and bony defects and/or alveolar injuries involving the loss of supporting bone are generally not replanted. For individuals with avulsed teeth with mature or closed apices who present within 2 h after injury, the tooth is placed in Hank's solution for about 30 min, then in doxycycline (1 mg/20 mL saline) to inhibit bacterial growth and aid pulpal revascularization; replantation and splinting with an acid-etch/resin splint for 7–10 days are then performed. Endodontic cleansing and shaping of the canal should be performed, and $Ca(OH)_2$ filling should be applied immediately prior to splint removal. The use of final gutta-percha obturation 6–12 months later is contingent on the resolution of canal and/or root pathology. To optimise the success of treatment, avulsed teeth should be replanted and stabilized within 2 h, before periodontal ligament cells become irreversibly necrotic. Teeth with apical openings >1 mm in diameter have a much better prognosis than do those with more mature or closed apices; however, when the extraoral period exceeds 2 h, apical root morphology has little effect on the treatment success rate.

4.4.3. Injuries to the supporting bone

Most alveolar fractures occur in the premolar and incisor regions. The treatment of these fractures involves proper reduction and rapid stabilization. Manipulation by pressure and rigid stabilization of the fragments are accepted closed-reduction techniques. Major displacement or difficulty with closed reduction may necessitate open reduction. Alignment of the involved teeth, edema of the segments, restoration of proper occlusion, and edema of the teeth in the fractured segment are important. The removal of teeth with no bony support may be considered, but should not be performed before the fractured bony segments have healed, even if the teeth are considered to be unsalvageable. Segment edema can be performed with acrylic or metal cap splints, orthodontic bands, fibreglass splints, transosseous wires, small or mini cortical plates, or transgingival lag screws; these materials should be applied for at least 4 weeks.

4.4.4. Complications

Pulp canal obliteration is characterized by the deposition of hard tissue within the root canal space and dark-yellow discolouration of the clinical crown. This complication is seen most frequently after tooth luxation or horizontal root fracture. A tooth with pulpal canal obliteration does not require treatment unless the pulp tissue becomes necrotic and develops periradicular radiolucency. Pulp necrosis is the most likely complication of dentoalveolar injury. Its incidence depends on the type and severity of injury and the extent of root development; teeth with fully formed roots are affected more often. If pulp necrosis is detected, root canal therapy should be initiated immediately to prevent inflammatory root resorption. Internal root resorption can be an issue after most dentoalveolar injuries. This process is usually detected radiographically; if it is identified at an early stage, root canal therapy has an excellent prognosis. The risk of tooth fracture after endodontic therapy is increased in cases of large defects. Follow-up radiography is useful for the detection of internal root resorption. If necrotic pulp is not removed, inflammation of the root surface may occur and the tooth root will be resorbed. Inflammatory root resorption can be detected radiographically and treated by $Ca(OH)_2$ dressing after canal debridement. Ankylosis can occur following damage to large areas of the periodontal membrane, as a primary result of trauma, or as a result of inflammatory root resorption. Osseous replacement proceeds slowly in adults; the tooth may serve for several years, but will loosen eventually.

5. Le Fort fractures

Rene Le Fort famously characterized the types of midfacial fracture caused by anteriorly directed forces [22-24] [Figure7-9]. Most Le Fort fractures are caused by motor vehicle accidents, and this type of trauma is often associated with other facial fractures and orthopaedic and neurologic injuries.

5.1. Clinical Examination

5.1.1. Le Fort I fractures (Guerin fracture)

In Le Fort I fractures, a horizontal fracture line separates the inferior portion of the maxilla, the horizontal plates of the palatal bones, and the inferior one-third of the sphenoid pterygoid processes from the superior two-thirds of the face, which remain associated with the skull. The entire maxillary dental arch may be mobile or wedged in a pathologic position. The patient may have an anterior open bite. Step deformities can be palpated intraorally if edema allows. Hematomas in the upper vestibule (Guerin's sign) and epistaxis may occur. Le Fort I fractures can be detected readily by orthopantomography, and CT provides a superior level of detail. [Figure 7].

5.1.2. Le Fort II fractures

In Le Fort II fractures, the pyramidal mid-face is separated from the rest of the facial skeleton and skull base. The fracture begins inferior to the nasofrontal suture and extends across the nasal bones and along the maxilla to the zygomaticomaxillary suture, including the inferomedial third of the orbit. The fracture then continues along the zygomaticomaxillary suture to and through the pterygoid plates. [Figure 8].

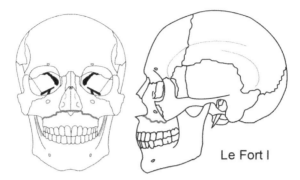

Figure 7. Le Fort I Fracture (Figure adapted from www.radiologytutorials.com)

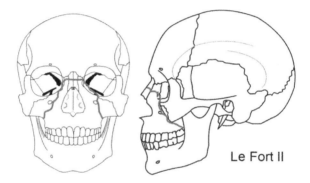

Figure 8. Le Fort II Fracture (Figure adapted from www.radiologytutorials.com)

5.1.3. Le Fort III fractures

In Le Fort III fractures, the face is essentially separated along the base of the skull due to force directed at the level of the orbit. The fracture line runs from the nasofrontal region along the medial orbit, through the superior and inferior orbital fissures, and then along the lateral orbital wall through the frontozygomatic suture. It then extends through the zygomaticotemporal suture and inferiorly through the sphenoid and the pterygomaxillary suture. In the past, Water's and lateral views were used to identify Le Fort fractures. CT and three-dimensional CT are now used most frequently, and axial and coronal scans are most useful for identifying midfacial fractures. Pterygoid plate fractures are found in all types of Le Fort fracture. Le Fort I fractures can be seen through the lateral aspect of the piriform aperture. Fractures of the infraorbital rim and zygomaticomaxillary buttress are unique to Le Fort II fractures. Only Le Fort III fractures involve the lateral orbital wall and zygomatic arch, and cerebrospinal fluid leakage can be a matter of concern. [Figure 9].

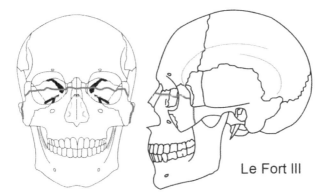

Le Fort III

Figure 9. Le Fort III Fracture (Figure adapted from www.radiologytutorials.com)

5.1.4. Treatment

The basic principle employed in the treatment of Le Fort fractures is fixation of the maxilla to the next highest stable structure, which differs with Le Fort fracture level. At the Le Fort I level, fixation is performed along the vertical buttresses of the maxilla at the piriform and zygomatic buttress. At higher Le Fort levels, fixation to the nasal bones, orbital rims, or zygomaticofrontal sutures may be necessary. The restoration of proper occlusion is a main goal of treatment. Reconstruction and fixation of the paranasal and zygomaticoalveolar buttresses are often sufficient to re-establish the proper position of the maxilla in Le Fort I fractures. Fractures with minimal or no displacement can heal spontaneously. Bleeding from the nasal wall or septal cracks is common and can be managed by various types of nasal packing. Tamponades can be used at other bleeding sites, such as those with lacerations or abrasions. Intermaxillary fixation with arch bars should be performed after reduction of the maxilla, followed by internal fixation of the maxillary vertical buttresses with plates and screws. Le Fort I fractures can generally be approached *via* maxillary vestibular incisions. Reduction of the maxilla can be challenging because of impaction, telescoping, or a significant interval of time between injury and treatment. If resistance is encountered during mobilisation of the maxilla, Rowe or Hayton–Williams disimpaction forceps may be used to help reduce the fracture [Figure 10,11].

Incomplete fractures may make maxillary mobilisation difficult; in such cases, completion of the fracture with osteotomies can facilitate reduction. In cases of severe comminution, inadequate dentition, periodontal disease, or edentulous arches (Gunning splints), fabricated occlusal or palatal splints can be applied to establish intermaxillary fixation.

Le Fort II fractures can be reduced with Rowe impaction forceps and intermaxillary fixation. A maxillary buccal vestibule incision and any of various approaches to the orbital rim can be used if open reduction is necessary. Bilateral Lynch incisions are to expose the nasofrontal suture [Figure 12].

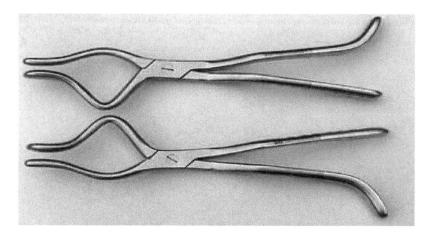

Figure 10. Rowe disimpaction forceps

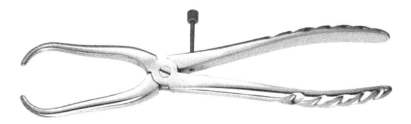

Figure 11. Hayton Williams forceps

Le Fort III fractures rarely occur in isolation and are usually components of panfacial fractures. Bicoronal incisions can be used to expose the naso-orbito-ethmoidal region, frontozygomatic sutures, and lateral orbital rims. Pre-auricular, lower lid, and maxillary vestibular incisions can be performed when necessary.

5.1.5. Complications

Patients who have undergone intermaxillary fixation may experience breathing problems, which can be resolved by opening the nasopharyngeal airways. Hemorrhage of the posterior superior alveolar artery should be suspected when perfuse bleeding occurs following any fracture of the posterior alveolar wall. Rapid decreases in blood pressure, hemoglobin, and hematocrit are other signs of fatal hemorrhage. If the artery cannot be ligated, embolization is indicated after the identification of the bleeding source *via* angiography. Some forms of trauma cause paranasal sinus fractures. Sinus complications, such as chronic sinusitis, polyps,

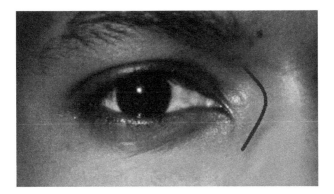

Figure 12. Lynch incision line

mucocele formation, and acute sinus infection may occur in such cases. Proper anatomic reduction of the sinuses can restore normal sinus function. Vision-related complications can be an issue before or after the reduction of a fracture, especially a high Le Fort fracture. Blindness, enophthalmos, and diplopia can occur due to intraorbital or retrobulbar hemorrhage or damage to the optic nerve caused by bone fragments. Improper rigid fixation of fracture segments will result in malocclusion; this complication usually occurs in patients with anterior open bites and/or class III fracture patterns. Improper rigid fixation may also cause numbness of the area innervated by the infraorbital nerve due to impingement of this nerve. A second surgical procedure is required to correct such complications. Malunion of maxillary fractures can obstruct the nasolacrimal ducts. Non-union of the segments may result in an inadequate blood supply, malpositioning, or infection. Foreign bodies, fractured teeth, and hematomas may cause infection.

6. Fractures of the zygomatic bone

Zygomatic bone fracture is the second most common midfacial injury, following nasal fracture. A zygomatic complex fracture is characterized by separation of the zygoma from its four articulations (frontal, sphenoidal, temporal, and maxillary). An independent fracture of the zygomatic arch is termed an isolated zygomatic arch fracture [Figure 13,14].

6.1. Clinical examination

The face is inspected and palpated to identify asymmetry caused by displaced fragments of the facial skeleton. Pain, ecchymosis, and periorbital edema with subconjunctival hemorrhage are the earliest clinical signs of a non-displaced zygomatic bone injury. Displaced fractures generally cause depression of the malar eminence and infraorbital rim. Damage to the zygomaticotemporal and infraorbital nerves may cause paraesthesia or anaesthesia in the cheek, lateral nose, upper lip, and maxillary anterior teeth. Epistaxis and diplopia are common

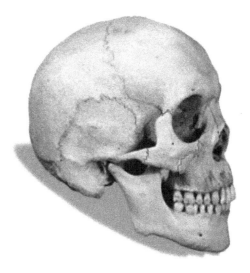

Figure 13. Zygomatic complex fracture

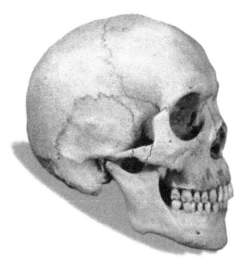

Figure 14. Isolated Zygomatic Arch fracture

in zygomatic bone fractures. Limitation of motion in the extraocular muscles and enophthal-mos or exophthalmos should be noted, as they can be signs of fracture of the orbital floor or medial or lateral orbital walls. In such cases, ophthalmologic consultation should be considered before surgical intervention. An isolated zygomatic arch fracture typically has an M-shaped pattern, with two fragments collapsed medially and often impinging on the masseter muscle or even the muscular process of the mandible. Medial displacement of the zygomatic arch may cause mandibular trismus as a result of masseter muscle spasm or mechanical impingement of the coronoid process against the displaced segments. Direct lateral force causes an isolated zygomatic arch fracture or an inferomedially displaced zygomatic complex fracture; frontal force usually produces an inferoposteriorly displaced fragment. Extraoral step deformities of the zygomatic arch and inferior and superolateral orbital margins, as well as intraoral step deformities of the zygomaticomaxillary buttress, may be palpable if the region is free of edema. Axial and coronal CT images inhibit visualisation of the buttress of the midfacial skeleton. Three-dimensional images may be used to obtain additional information about the relationships of displaced and rotated fractured segments to surrounding bony structures. Plain radiography employing Waters' and Caldwell's views can also be used to detect zygomatic complex fractures. The submentovertex view is very helpful for the evaluation of the zygomatic arch and malar projection.

6.2. Treatment

The management of zygomatic bone fractures depends on the degree of displacement and the resultant aesthetic and functional deficits. Surgery can be delayed until the majority of facial edema is gone. Isolated zygomatic arch and zygomatic complex fractures with minimal or no displacement are not managed surgically. A soft diet restriction can help to avoid secondary fracture displacement. When displacement and minimal comminution are present, the Gillies technique is the standard reduction treatment for isolated zygomatic arch fractures [Figure 15]. In the Gillies approach, a 2-cm-long temporal incision is made behind the hairline, and the subcutaneous and superficial temporal fascia are dissected to the level of the temporalis muscle to reach the underlying temporal surface of the zygomatic bone; a zygomatic elevator is then used to reduce the arch fracture [25]. The use of a J-shaped hook elevator through a periauricular incision made anterior to the articular eminence and inferior to the zygomatic arch is an alternative approach for reducing zygomatic arch fractures. This approach is faster than the Gillies approach, but it can easily cause damage to the frontal branches of the facial nerve. Fixation of zygomatic arch fractures can be performed by packing the temporal fossa or using transcutaneous circumzygomatic arch wires while providing support with metal or aluminium finger splints. Open reduction is rarely performed in highly comminuted zygomatic arch fractures because it requires a time-consuming coronal incision.

Displaced zygomatic complex fractures require open reduction and internal fixation. Miniplates and microplates provide the best results with minimal complications. A useful option for displaced zygomatic fractures is the application of a transcutaneous Carroll–Girard screw in the malar region [Figure 16].

This technique enables excellent manipulation of the fractured segment for reduction. Reduction of the frontozygomatic suture, zygomaticomaxillary buttress, and inferior orbital rim should be the main goal of the treatment protocol. The perfect reduction of these three points of reference allows proper positioning of the fractured segment. The location and

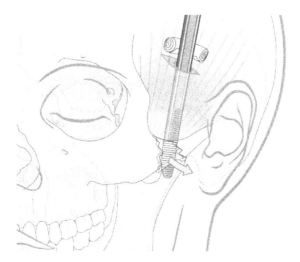

Figure 15. Gillies approach to zygomatic arch (Figure adapted from www.aofoundation.org)

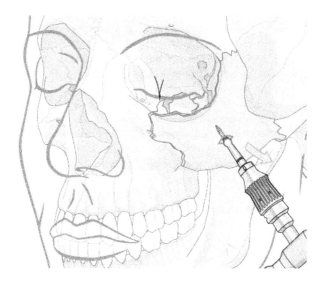

Figure 16. Useof Carroll-Girard screw (Figure adapted from www.aofoundation.org)

number of fixation sites depend on the fracture pattern, location, direction of displacement, and degree of instability. In more severe fractures, perfect reduction can be achieved with the use of the zygomatic arch as a fourth reference point. The zygomaticomaxillary buttress should be reduced first *via* an intraoral approach, while this structure is easy to reach; this technique leaves no scar and may achieve reduction of the entire fractured segment. The zygomatico-maxillary buttress is approached surgically through a 3–5-mm-long incision in the maxillary vestibule above the mucogingival junction, extending from the canine region to first molar region. The protocol for minimally comminuted and displaced fractures should be temporary edema of the zygomaticofrontal suture with wires, reduction of the zygomaticomaxillary buttress and inferior orbital rim, and then replacement of the temporary zygomaticofrontal edema with a plate. The zygomaticofrontal suture is approached surgically through a lateral eyebrow incision, and the inferior orbital rim is approached *via* subciliary and transconjunctival incisions [Figure 17-19].

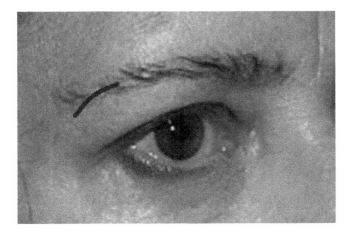

Figure 17. Lateral eyebrow incision line

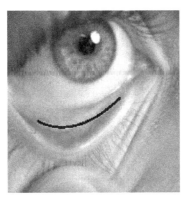

Figure 18. Transconjuctival incision line

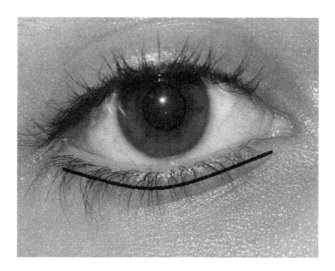

Figure 19. Subciliary incision line

In complex and highly comminuted fractures, the zygomatic arch should be reconstructed first; a coronal flap is usually used to gain access to this structure.

6.3. Complications

Restoration of the natural contour of the zygoma is the key to restoring facial projection in patients with displaced and comminuted fractures. Inadequate flattening the zygomatic arch and failure to achieve optimal rotation of the zygomaticomaxillary complex result in malar eminence flattening, asymmetry, and widening of the face. Inadequate reduction or edema of segments may cause malunion.

Poor or excessive reconstruction of the orbital rim should be avoided because an increase in orbital volume can cause enophthalmos and a decrease can cause exophthalmos. Diplopia can be caused by edema, hematoma, injury to cranial nerves 3, 4, or 6, and damage to extraocular muscles, and may heal spontaneously except in the latter case.

Although damage to the zygomaticomaxillary and zygomaticofacial nerves is less common, zygomaticomaxillary complex fractures often cause damage to the infraorbital foramen. Anaesthesia of the lower eyelid and malar and upper lip areas is common in infraorbital nerve injuries. Proper reduction of the fractured segments usually minimizes the risk of permanent symptoms. Blindness immediately after surgery may indicate impingement of the orbital apex contents by a bony fragment. Retrobulbar hematomas rarely develop, but compression of the central retinal artery causing disruption of the retinal circulation may lead to irreversible ischaemia of the optic nerve and permanent blindness.

Patients with zygomatic fractures may suffer from trismus, which may be caused by impingement of the zygomatic bone on the coronoid process of the mandible or ankylosis of the coronoid process to the zygomatic arch. If a previous zygomatic bone or arch fracture has been reduced improperly, the zygomatic bone should be repositioned *via* osteotomy; otherwise, coronoidectomy is the most common solution.

7. Orbital fractures

Isolated orbital fracture is not a common type of midfacial fracture, but the incidence of midfacial fractures involving the orbit is high because all Le Fort II and III fractures and those of the naso-orbito-ethmoidal and zygomaticomaxillary complexes involve orbital injury. Orbital fractures may affect the internal and/or external orbital frame. Thus, fractures of the orbital region can be discussed in the context of zygomaticomaxillary complex, naso-orbito-ethmoidal complex, and isolated orbital fractures.

7.1. Clinical examination

As discussed above, zygomaticomaxillary complex fracture is the most common fracture type with orbital involvement. Like naso-orbito-ethmoidal fractures (discussed below), zygomaticomaxillary complex fractures are caused by blunt force applied directly to the bone. Isolated fractures of the orbit often occur as a result of direct force to the globe of the eye. A sudden increase in intraorbital pressure creates an outward force that causes fracture of the weakest bony structures in internal orbital walls. Isolated orbital fractures can be classified as 'blow-out' or 'blow-in'. Most blow-out fractures affect the anteroinferomedial aspect of the orbital cavity and displace the orbital globe posteromedially and inferiorly. A significant increase in the volume of the orbital cavity results in enophthalmos of the globe. Herniation of the orbital roof and globe to the maxillary sinus occurs in such fractures. When an isolated fracture is caused by low-energy force, linear fracture of the orbit may be detected. Linear fractures retain periosteal attachments and do not cause orbital globe herniation to the maxillary sinus or complete perforation of the maxillary sinus roof. More severe trauma causes a complex fracture involving two or more orbital walls. In complex internal orbital fractures, the globe is often displaced posteriorly and the optic canal may be involved. Blow-in fractures affect the orbital roof and may be diagnosed after severe injury of the anterior skull base. Rupture of the orbital roof reduces the orbital volume and often causes anteroinferior globe displacement.

The affected region should be inspected carefully to identify the presence of edema, chemosis, ecchymosis, lacerations, ptosis, asymmetric lid drape, canalicular injury, and/or canthal tendon disruption. Any step deformity or mobility around the orbital rim should be palpated before edema develops in surrounding tissues. Neurosensation of the infraorbital and supraorbital nerves should be tested. Ophthalmologic consultation is very important and necessary. Limitation of ocular movements can be caused by mechanical entrapment or neurologic injury. Three-dimensional CT and magnetic resonance imaging are preferred for the evaluation of orbital fractures. Waters' projection is the most useful plain radiographic modality because it enables visualisation of the orbital floor and roof. Ophthalmic ultrasonography and color Doppler imaging can provide additional information.

7.2. Treatment

Subciliary and transconjunctival incisions are the most aesthetically acceptable approaches to the orbital floor. Linear injuries of the orbital floor require no intervention unless they show signs of soft-tissue entrapment in fractured but self-reduced sites. In patients with blow-out or blow-in fractures, soft- and hard-tissue reduction and reconstruction are necessary. Grafting of the injured site with autografts, allografts, or alloplastic materials may be necessary to achieve proper anatomic reduction and stability and to prevent soft-tissue contraction. The iliac crest and nasal septal cartilage are the best donor sites for autografts, and the use of alloplastic titanium mesh can be successful in cases requiring extra support.

7.3. Complications

Most internal orbital fractures cause volumetric contraction or expansion of the orbital cavity, which may lead to diplopia, enophthalmos, exophthalmos, proptosis, and/or extraocular muscle imbalance. Extraocular muscle imbalance and diplopia can be the result of extraocular muscle entrapment or neuropathy of the 3rd to 5th cranial nerves. An increase in orbital volume causes enophthalmos, which may occur weeks or months after injury.

For some challenging fractures of the orbital floor, the transconjunctival approach may be safer than other methods. The placement of a transconjunctival incision at the conjunctival fornix appears to minimize the risk of eyelid malposition. A transantral endoscopic approach is an alternative method that avoids potential damage caused by lower-lid incisions.

8. Naso-orbito-ethmoidal fractures

Naso-orbito-ethmoidal facture can occur either in isolation or in association with other midfacial fractures. Most associated injuries affect the cervical spine and ocular and intracranial regions. This fracture type is caused by focused high-energy transfer to the intercanthal area. Because the naso-orbito-ethmoidal area contains several types of tissue (bone, cartilage, tendons, ocular tissue) restoration is challenging.

8.1. Clinical examination

Naso-orbito-ethmoidal fractures are characterized by three major post-injury symptoms: increased intercanthal distance, diminished nasal projection, and impaired nasofrontal and lacrimal drainage.

Markowitz et al. [26] developed the most widely used classification system for naso-orbito-ethmoidal fractures, which distinguishes three fracture types [Figure 20]:

• Type I: the medial canthal tendon is attached to a single, large central fragment

• Type II: the medial canthal tendon is attached to a comminuted but manageable central fragment; the canthal tendon remains attached to a fragment that is sufficiently large to allow osteosynthesis

- Type III: the medial canthal tendon is attached to a comminuted and unmanageable central fragment; the fragments are either too small to allow osteosynthesis or completely detached.

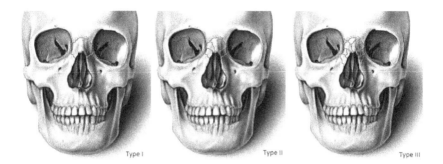

Figure 20. Classification of Nasoorbitoethmoidal fractures

Periorbital ecchymosis, subconjunctival hemorrhage, and pain are the most common signs and symptoms of naso-orbito-ethmoidal fractures. Other signs and symptoms include skin and mucosal lacerations, epistaxis, nasal obstruction, edema, telecanthus, and increased canthal angles. Depression of the bony segment causes internal and external nasal cosmetic deformities. Edema may obscure such depression for up to 5 days, and most surgeons recommend the postponement of surgery until the edema has resolved. The impaction of bony segments to the orbit may cause exophthalmos, proptosis, or ptosis. Fractures of cribriform plate and posterior wall of the frontal sinus may cause cerebrospinal fluid leakage. Nasal bone mobility, traumatic telecanthus, crepitus, and depressibility of the area are the clinical digital-examination findings for naso-orbito-ethmoidal fractures.

Increased intercanthal distance, termed telecanthus, is a key deformity resulting from naso-orbito-ethmoidal injury. Normal intercanthal distances are 29–36 mm in males and 29–34 mm in females; a distance exceeding 40 mm is classified as telecanthus and may indicate that surgical treatment is required.The medial canthal tendon is a very important anatomic factor in naso-orbito-ethmoidal injuries resulting in telecanthus. The pretarsal portions of the orbicularis oculi muscle in the upper and lower lids unite at the canthus to form the medial canthal tendon. The superficial portion of this tendon provides support to the eyelids and maintains the integrity of the palpebral fissure. Restoration of this component after canthal detachment is critical for maintaining proper eyelid appearance. The deeper portion, also called Horner's muscle, attaches to the posterior lacrimal crest and assists in the movement of fluid through the lacrimal system. Disruption of the medial canthal tendon causes contraction of the orbicularis oculi muscle, increasing the intercanthal distance and laterally displacing the rounded contour of the medial palpebral fissure. The 'bowstring test' is a useful method of assessing the status of the medial canthal tendon's attachment to the bone. This test involves lateral pulling of the lid while palpating the tendon area to detect movement of fracture segments [27] [Figure 21].

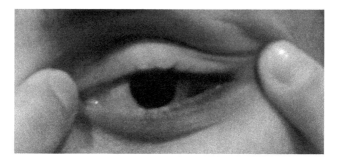

Figure 21. Bowstring test

Two- and three-dimensional CT using axial and coronal views are the most valuable imaging methods for the diagnosis of naso-orbito-ethmoidal fractures. The use of conventional imaging techniques is not recommended because these modalities do not provide adequate information.

8.2. Treatment

The goals of naso-orbito-ethmoidal fracture treatment are the resolution of the three major issues described above: Establishment of proper nasal projection, narrowing of the intercanthal distance, and establishment of the nasofrontal and lacrimal fluid route. The surgeon should seek to achieve satisfactory results in a single surgery because corrective secondary surgery may cause scarring and fibrosis. For this reason, most authors have advocated the postponement of surgery for 3–7 days to allow for the recession of edema. For naso-orbito-ethmoidal fractures involving a single fragment (type I), treatment can be attempted with closed reduction and the provision of intranasal packing support. If the fragment cannot be reduced satisfactorily by closed reduction, the operation should be converted immediately to an open reduction to avoid the need for secondary surgery. In most cases, a transoral approach is sufficient to reach the injured area without an additional incision.

Proper restoration of types II and III naso-orbito-ethmoidal fractures usually require wide access, which can be provided only by a coronal flap. Wide exposure of the nasal bones and medial orbital walls can be achieved readily. When necessary, a transoral approach can be used to access the paranasal areas and a transconjunctival approach can be used to expose the inferior orbital rim or inferomedial wall. Existing lacerations can also be used to access the injured area. Transcutaneous approaches are not considered to be acceptable because they cause facial scarring.

In severe naso-orbito-ethmoidal injuries, nasal dorsal strut grafting is often required to re-establish support for the entire nose. This graft is cantilevered from the stable frontal bone and placed in the subcutaneous plane, extending inferiorly to the nasal tip.

When the medial canthal tendon is detached completely or attached to an unusable bone fragment, its proper position must be secured immediately using medial canthopexy. The medial canthal tendon should be reduced into a position slightly posterosuperior to the posterior lacrimal crest. The tendon is then sutured with a wire passing transnasally to a cantilevered miniplate on the opposing (undamaged) side. The canthopexy should be positioned sufficiently deep in the orbit to achieve the proper shape of the palpebral fissure and lower lid, as the superficial portion of the medial canthal tendon secures the position of the lower lid and contour of the palpebral fissure. Proper positioning of the medial canthal tendon will achieve correct lacrimal fluid drainage, which is aided by the deep portion of the tendon. When nasofrontal obstruction is a concern, endoscopic frontal sinus surgery can be indicated to re-establish nasofrontal drainage. The medial canthal tendon should be slightly over-reduced in canthopexy procedures to compensate for remodelling of related tissues.

8.3. Complications

Cosmetic deformities are foreseeable after nasal and naso-orbito-ethmoidal injuries. Postoperative septal hematoma, septal abscess, and/or destructive fracture of the septal cartilage/bone are the postoperative causes of nasal deformity. Massive comminution of the naso-orbito-ethmoidal complex is classically associated with saddle nose deformity. Bone grafting is required in most patients to establish proper nasal projection, symmetry, and contour. However, even bone grafts can be associated with potential resorption problems in the long term. Depending on the fracture level, cartilage or bone grafts and nasal implants can be used to improve the appearance of these deformities.

Septal deviation due to inadequate closed reduction often results in external nasal asymmetry. Direct septal visualisation *via* the open rhinoplasty approach is preferred for the correction of this defect.

After naso-orbito-ethmoidal injury, scar contracture results in cosmetic and functional deformities. Thus, secondary surgery should be avoided because it may result in scarring.

Open reduction and internal fixation procedures often damage the medial canthal tendon or nasolacrimal apparatus. As a result, epiphora related to nasolacrimal duct obstruction can be an issue. Intubation or stenting of the lacrimal duct may be necessary in such cases.

9. Midfacial fractures in children

Midfacial fractures are not common in children; they account for only 1–8% of pediatric fractures [28-31] and usually affect the mandible. This low incidence is related to the protection provided by the mandible and cranium, which absorb most of the traumatic impact, and to the elastic nature of midfacial bones and flexibility of osseous suture lines [32]. Children form a distinct patient group in maxillofacial surgery due to significant differences between the facial skeletons of children and adults. Depending on the patient's age, these differences include small bone size, small paranasal sinus volume, growth potential, the presence of tooth germs in alveoli during primary and mixed dentition stages, a more rapid healing process compared with adults, and difficulty with cooperation resulting in the need for general anaesthesia in more cases than in adults [33]. The proportion of children in whom midfacial fractures are identified has increased over time, probably due to the increased use of adequate imaging modalities [34]. CT has largely supplanted standard radiography as the preferred imaging method for pediatric facial trauma.

The presence of tooth germs in alveoli potentially creates zones of weakness in the jaws and limits the placement of certain plate and screw types, given the need to avoid damage to the developing dentition. The treatment of pediatric patients with midfacial fractures using intermaxillary fixation is also quite difficult, and erupting or exfoliating teeth can be an issue. On the other hand, the on-going processes of tooth eruption and exfoliation may compensate for minor inaccuracies in reduction and fixation. Recognition of the differences between children and their adult counterparts is important in facial rehabilitation.

Several aspects of dentoalveolar trauma management in children differ from that in adults. Developing roots have open apices, and the preservation of pulp vitality is important. In complicated crown and crown–root fractures, pulpotomy can be performed 1–2 mm below the exposed pulp tissue and $Ca(OH)_2$ or mineral trioxide aggregate can be applied. The second step in such cases is composite restoration or bonding of the crown fragment to the tooth. If the pulp is necrotic, apexification with intracanal application of $Ca(OH)_2$ must be used instead of pulpotomy. In pediatric cases of intrusion, spontaneous re-eruption may occur. Orthodontic repositioning can be a second treatment plan unless movement is observed within about 3 weeks. In the pediatric dentition, osseous replacement in ankylosis occurs much faster than in adults; dentoalveolar ankylosis usually interferes with alveolar process growth, and the tooth might be malpositioned.

Fractures in the maxillary region tend to be less comminuted in children than in adults because children's paranasal sinuses are not fully developed. Open reduction and internal fixation are the preferred treatment methods, but intermaxillary fixation may be necessary in some cases. Avoiding damage to permanent tooth germs is a mandatory indication for closed reduction. Intermaxillary fixation with arch bars presents some difficulties in patients with mixed dentition, but the fixation period can be shorter than in adults. Teeth may be avulsed by the force of arch bars, and the fixation of arch bars to the teeth may not provide adequate retention because of weak and undeveloped roots. For this reason, the fabrication and use of Gunning splints to provide retention from the zygomatic arches, piriform apertures, and mandible *via* circumferential wires is recommended when intermaxillary fixation is necessary. As in adults, restoration of the normal anatomic position of the midfacial skeleton in children generally requires open reduction and stable fixation with miniplates and screws. In pediatric Le Fort II and III fractures, open reduction and internal fixation are necessary to re-establish proper anatomic and functional relationships. Pediatric fractures in the maxillary region are often of the greenstick type, which increases the complexity of fragment reduction. Because a greenstick fracture line limits fragment movement, proper reduction may require osteotomy.

Paediatric orbital fractures resulting in herniation and extraocular muscle entrapment require immediate intervention and even orbital exploration. Fractures of the orbital floor or wall in children heal rapidly, increasing the risks of scar cicatrisation and related ischemic necrosis of entrapped tissues.

Because the development of the nasal septum is a very important factor in facial growth, post-traumatic septal hematoma, which may cause septal necrosis and resorption, should not be ignored because it may result in saddle nose deformity.

Author details

Sertac Aktop*, Onur Gonul, Tulin Satilmis, Hasan Garip and Kamil Goker

Department of Oral and Maxillofacial Surgery, Marmara University, Istanbul, Turkey

References

[1] Gassner R, Tuli T, Hachl O, Rudisch A, Ulmer H. Cranio-Maxillofacial Trauma: A 10 Year Review Of 9543 Cases With 21 067 İnjuries. Journal Of Cranio-Maxillofacial Surgery. 2003;31:51–61

[2] Thomas DW, Hill CM: Etiology And Changing Patterns Of Maxillofacial Trauma. In: Booth PW, Schendel SA, Hausamen JE (Eds) Maxillofacial Surgery, Vol. Churchill Livingstone, 3, 2000

[3] Mouzakes J, Koltai PJ, Kuhar S, Bernstein DS, Wing P, Salsberg E:The İmpact Of Airbags And Seat Belts On The İncidence And Severity Of Maxillofacial İnjuries İn Automobile Accidents İn New York State. Arch Otolaryngol – Head Neck Surg. 2001;127:1189–1193

[4] Cook H E, Rowe M. A Retrospective Study Of 356 Midfacial Fractures Occurring İn 225 Patients. J Oral Maxillolac Surg. 1990;48:574 578

[5] Girotto JA, Mackenzie E, Fowler C, Redett R, Robertson B, Manson PN:Long-Term Physical İmpairment And Functional Outcomes After Complex Facial Fractures. Plast Reconstr Surg. 2001;108:312–327

[6] Afzelius LE, Rosen C: Facial Fractures: A Review Of 368 Cases. Int J Oral Surg. 1980;9:25

[7] Motamedi M H K. An Assessment Of Maxillofacial Fractures: A 5-Year Study Of 237 Patients. J Oral Maxillofac Surg. 2003;61:61-64

[8] Ansari M H. Maxillofacial Fractures İn Hamedan Province, Iran: A Retrospective Study (1987–2001).Journal Of Cranio-Maxillofacial Surgery. 2004;32, 28–34

[9] Thorén H, Snäll J, Salo J, Taipale L S, Kormi E, Lindqvist C,Törnwall J. Occurrence And Types Of Associated Injuries İn Patients With Fractures Of The Facial Bones. J Oral Maxillofac Surg. 2010;68:805-810

[10] Banks P, Brown A: Etiology, Surgical Anatomy And Classification. In: Banks P, Brown A (Eds), Fractures Of The Facial Skeleton. Philadelphia, USA: Elsevier, 1e4, 2001

[11] Shankar A N Et Al.. The Pattern Of The Maxillofacial Fractures E A Multicentre Retrospective Study. Journal Of Cranio-Maxillo-Facial Surgery Xxx (2012) 1-5 Doi: 10.1016/J.Jcms.2011.11.004

[12] Simpson DA, Mclean AJ: Mechanisms Of İnjury. In: David DJ, Simpson DA (Eds) Craniomaxillofacial Trauma, Vol. 101. Churchill Livingstone, 1995

[13] Killey H C. Fractures Of The Middle Third Of The Facial Skeleton. Bristol: John Wright & Sons Limited, 1977

[14] Norton N S. Netter's Head And Neck Anatomy For Dentistry. Philadelphia: Saunders Elsevier, 2007

[15] Teasdale G, Jennett B. Assessment of coma and impaired consciousness: a practical scale. Lancet 1974;2:81–4.

[16] Z. Nya´ra´dy, E. Orsi, K. Nagy, L. Olasz, J. Nya´ra´dy: Transgingival lag-screw osteosynthesis of alveolar process fracture. Int. J. Oral Maxillofac. Surg. 2010; 39: 779–782.

[17] Ellis E III. Soft Tissue and Dentoalveolar Injuries. In: Hupp J R et al. (ed.). Contemporary Oral and Maxillofacial Surgery Fifth Edition. Missouri: Mosby Elsevier; 2008. p474-7

[18] Fonseca RJ, Marciani RD, Hendler BH. Oral and maxillofacial surgery, trauma. Vol 3. Diagnosis and management of dentoalveolar injuries. Philadelphia (PA):W.B. Saunders Co; 2000. p. 48–50.

[19] Snawder KD, Bastawni AE, O'Toole TJ. Tooth fragments lodged in unexpected areas. JAMA 1976;233:1378–9.

[20] Leather D L, Gowans R E. Management of Alveolar and Dental Fractures, In: Miloro M (ed.) Peterson's Principles of Oral and Maxillofacial Surgery Second Edition. London: BC Decker Inc; 2004; 383-400.

[21] Andreasen JO, editor. Traumatic injuries of the teeth. 1st ed. Philadelphia (PA): W.B. Saunders; 1972.

[22] Le Fort R. Etude experimentale sur les fractures de la machoire superiore. Rev Chir 1901; 23:208–27.

[23] Le Fort R. Etude experimentale sur les fractures de la machoire superiore. Rev Chir 1901;23:360–79.

[24] Le Fort R. Etude experimentale sur les fractures de la machoire superiore. Rev Chir 1901;23:479–507.

[25] Gillies HD, Kilner TP, Stone D. Fractures of the malarzygomatic compound, with a description of a new x-ray position. Br J Surg 1927;14:651.

[26] Markowitz BL, Manson PN, Sargent L, et al. Management of medial canthal tendon in nasoethmoid orbital fractures: the importance of the central fragment in classification and treatment, Plast Reconstr Surg. 1991;87:843-853

[27] Furnas DW, Dircoll MJ. Eyelash traction test to determine if the medial canthal ligament is detached. Plast Reconstr Surg 1973;52:315–7.

[28] Rowe NL. Fractures of the jaws of children. J Oral Surg. 1969;27:497-507

[29] Posnick JC, Wells M, Pron GE. Pediatric facial fractures: evolving paterns of treatment. J Oral Maxillofac Surg. 1993;51:836-844

[30] Gassner R, Tuli T, Höchl O, et al. Craniomaxillofacial trauma in children: a review of 3385 cases with 6060 injuries in 10 years. J Oral Maxillofac Surg. 2004;62:399-407

[31] Qaqish C, Caccamese Jr JF. Pediatric Mid-face Fractures. In: Bagheri SC, Bell RB, Khan HA (ed.). Current therapy in oral and maxillofacial surgery. Missouri: Saunders Elsevier; 2012.p851-8

[32] Ferreira P, Marques M, Pinho C, Rodrigues J, Reis J, Amarante J. Midfacial fractures in children and adolescents: a review of 492 cases. British Journal of Oral and Maxillofacial Surgery. 2004;42:501−505

[33] Iatrou I, Theologie-Lygidakis N, Tzerbos F. Surgical Protocols And Outcome For The Treatment Of Maxillofacial Fractures İn Children: 9 Years' Experience. Journal Of Cranio-Maxillo-Facial Surgery. 2010;38:511-516

[34] Thorén H, Iso-Kungas P, Iizuka T, Lindqvist C, Törnwall J. Changing trends in causes and patterns of facial fractures in children Oral Surg Oral Med Oral Pathol Oral Radiol Endod. 2009;107:318-324.

Chapter 2

Management of Mandibular Fractures

Amrish Bhagol, Virendra Singh and Ruchi Singhal

Additional information is available at the end of the chapter

1. Introduction

The treatment of mandibular fractures has been in a constant state of evolution over the past few decades. The most significant advancements related to the management of fractures of the mandible are based on specific technical refinements in the methods of internal fixation. Also there is improvement in the knowledge of anatomy, pathophysiology, pharmacology and biomaterial science which influence our current management of mandibular fractures. Recent mandibular fracture management techniques have allowed for decreased infection rates and biological stable fixation of bone segments. This philosophy produces bony union and restoration of preinjury occlusion and normally eliminates the need for wire maxillomandibular immobilization. All this adds up to a faster, safer, more comfortable return to function. In spite of the presence of these modern techniques, closed reduction has by no means fallen by the wayside and still remains a commonly used procedure.This chapter presents an overview of general treatment principles in the management of mandibular fractures and also discusses the treatment strategies in detail depending on the age and anatomical site involved (symphysis, angle, condyle etc). Mandibular fractures in children and adults need different treatment approaches. Similarly, fractures of different anatomical sites in the mandible need different treatment modalities; they differ in their biomechanics, treatment requirements and complications. So each fracture is discussed individually taking care of the different schools of thought and controversies regarding their management. Major advances in the treatment of mandibular fracture in terms of biomaterials and minimally invasive surgical techniques are also discussed.

2. Historical overview

Historical references to mandible fracture diagnosis and treatment date back to 1650 BC as evidenced by the Edwin Smith Surgical Papyrus.[1,2] The patient described subsequently died, likely from infection secondary to the mandibular fracture. Hippocrates, the "father of medicine," also described the treatment of mandible fractures with circumferential dental wiring in some of his initial writings.[3] However, it was Salicetti, in 1275, who first present-ed maxillomandibular fixation as a treatment for fractures of the mandibles,[4,5] ; the reader was advised to "tie the teeth of the uninjured jaw to the teeth of the injured jaw." Although a fundamental concept in contemporary facial fracture management, Salicetti's concept of MMF disappeared for centuries until Gilmer applied the technique clinically and described its utility in more detail in the United States in 1887.[6] Despite a few early attempts at rigid internal fixation, for most of the 20th century[7], the management of mandibular and maxil-lary fractures was limited to the application of bandages, maxillomandibular fixation or Gunning-type splints for the edentulous. Later external frames were used in combination with pin fixation. Fracture treatment by open approach and direct transosseous wiring was avoided in the preantibiotic era since it almost inevitably produced infection and osteomye-litis. It was reserved for use in select cases involving the posterior mandible (i.e. ramus/ angle) or in edentulous patients. The earliest reports of mandibular fractures treated with an open reduction were from Buck, using an iron loop, and Kinlock, using a silver wire. [8,9] Gilmer, in 1881, described the use of two heavy rods placed on either side of the fracture that were wired together.[10] Schede (circa 1888) is credited with the first use of a true bone plate made of steel and secured with four screws.[9] In the 1960s, Luhr developed the vitalli-um mandibular compression plate through his research on rigid fixation of the facial skele-ton. Luhr and Spiessl reintroduced the idea of utilizing miniature bone plates in the repair of mandibular fractures in 1968 and 1972.[11] In 1976, Spiessl and others continued to advance techniques of open reduction and internal fixation (ORIF) and developed the principles now advocated by the Arbeitsgemeinschaft fur Osteosynthesefragen (Association for Osteosyn-thesis/Association for the Study of Internal Fixation (AO/ ASIF).[12] This concept was un-fortunately based on trying to 'fit' orthopedic principles and, worse, orthopaedic materials to the complex structures of the facial skeleton. The belief was that callus formation repre-sented a failure of the healing process, because of excessive and undesirable movements across the fracture. Thus more heavy and complex methods were devised to increase the sta-bility across the fracture. These plates were bulky, difficult to use and always required large skin incisions. This philosophy failed to see that perfectly good reduction and healing could be achieved by very unstable fixation methods like wiring of the teeth together. Whilst man-dibular maxillary wire fixation was potentially dangerous and unpleasant, it was very effec-tive in healing bones. These crude, heavy plating systems did, however, demonstrate the benefits of avoiding wire maxillomandibular fixation, including comfort, return to normal mastication and normal oral function. In reality, these heavy compression plates had a high morbidity. The neck scars were undesirable, nerve damage to both the facial and inferior al-veolar nerves was common and infection of the plates frequent; a second operation to re-move the plates was always necessary. The principles of heavy compression plating could not be applied to the thin bones of the upper facial skeleton.

One useful technique to arise from this principle of applying orthopedic material to the fa-cial skeleton was the use of lag screws, which is a simple technique of producing interfrag-mentary stability by compression. These have a large screw hole bored on the outer fragment and allow the tightening of the screw to compress the fragments together. In a few sites in the mandible it can be a simple effective treatment via the intraoral approach but since the screw must cross the fracture at right angles it has limited use. In the 1970s another concept of internal fixation for the repair of mandibular fractures was introduced by Michelet and colleagues and refined by Champy and co-workers; they placed small, bendable, noncompression plates along the lines of ideal osteosynthesis.[13,14] Both of these techniques have proven to be effective and are routinely used in the contemporary management of mandibular fractures. The use of small miniplates was successfully integrated into the rest of the facial skeleton, being refined and miniaturized for the periorbital and cranial non-load bearing areas. Most recently, bone-plating systems made from resorbable polymer have been introduced. Although these materials show significant promise, they have been utilized most often in the non-load bearing cranial and orbital regions. The resorbable materials themselves and the techniques used in their application continue to be redefined at a rapid pace in this early phase of development.[15,16]

3. Diagnosis

The diagnosis of mandibular fractures must begin with a careful history and clinical examination. Immediate attention must always be given to problems associated with airway compromise and bleeding which may endanger the patient's life. Once the airway, breathing and circulation have been adequately assessed, a quick neurologic function evaluation should be performed. Standard trauma protocols such as those described in the Advanced Trauma Life Support guidelines from the American College of Surgeons should be utilized for a comprehensive evaluation. While taking history, information about the mode of injury will often suggest a specific fracture pattern and may provide the surgeon with valuable insight regarding the potential for concomitant injuries. Patients who sustain fractures involving the mandible will often report a paresthesia or change in their occlusion noted immediately after the traumatic event. The patient's past medical and surgical history, medication use and known drug allergies should also be reviewed. Temporomandibular joint dysfunction and any previous non-surgical or surgical treatment should be carefully documented. When a mandibular fracture is suspected, meticulous clinical examination of the maxillofacial region is critical and should be carried out prior to the ordering of radiographic imaging studies.

3.1. Clinical examination

Without question, a change in occlusion is the most common physical finding in patients with fractures of the mandible. When examining the occlusion, it is important to consider that the patient may have had an abnormal dental or skeletal occlusal relationship (Class II or Class III) prior to the injury. Changes in occlusion will likely accompany fractures of the mandible, but may also be present in soft tissue trauma of the TMJ, fractures of the alveolus, dental fractures or fractures of the maxilla. When the fracture traverses a region of the mandible that includes the inferior alveolar nerve, some level of neurosensory disturbance involving this nerve will result. Abnormalities in the mandibular range of motion or deviation of the mandible are also indicative of fracture, as can be an inability to close completely. These restrictions may also be the result of internal TMJ injury or hematoma. Sublingual ecchymosis is highly suggestive of a fracture involving the mandibular arch. Another indication of fracture is a bony step which is most easily recognized by careful palpation along the inferior border of the mandible.

3.2. Radiographic examination

Proper treatment of fractures of the mandible is dependent on proper diagnosis of the injury. Paramount in diagnosis of the details of the fracture and therefore the treatment options is the radiographic evaluation. In principle, these should be at least two films taken at right angles to each other. The plain films used include oblique views, posteroanterior (PA) Towne's view, and possibly a lateral view. All institutions have these views available to them. Some continue to use these views for routine screening of mandibular trauma. The efficacy of these views remains controversial if other screening techniques are available. Because of the diagnostic efficacy of panoramic radiographs and CT, the surgeons at our institution seldom obtain plain views except for the Towne's view, which we have found to be very useful in assessing displacement of subcondylar fractures.

A diagnostic-quality panoramic radiograph is the most comprehensive view possible with a single film and allows satisfactory visualization of all regions of the mandible (condyle, ramus, body and symphysis).[17] It is also useful in examining the existing dentition, presence of impacted teeth with respect to the fracture, alveolar process and position of the mandibular canal. [Figure 1]

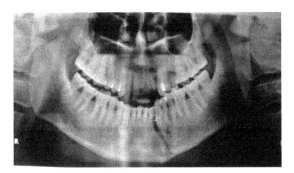

Figure 1. Panoramic tomogram showing parasymphysis and subcondylar fractures of mandible.

In situations where a panoramic view of the mandible is not available, a series of different views of the mandible is required to adequately view all the anatomic regions of interest. This is more labor intensive and costly and subjects the patient to a higher dose of radiation. Despite the good visualization of the dentoalveolar structures obtained by a panoramic radiograph, additional periapical or occlusal radiographs are often helpful in viewing specific areas of concern with more detail, especially when tooth or alveolar fractures are suspected. Parasymphysis fractures often benefit from occlusal films to display any obliquity of the fracture, which will certainly change the fixation method.

3.3. Computed tomography examination

Computed tomography *(CT)* currently offers the most detailed and comprehensive view of the facial skeleton. Current protocols allow for axial, coronal and reconstructed three-dimensional images to be formulated [Figure 2].

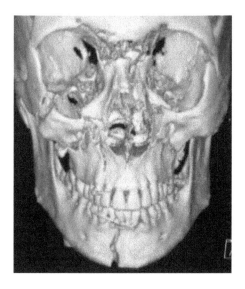

Figure 2. Three dimensional reconstruction CT of a panfacial fracture.

Despite this superior three-dimensional visualization, the use of CT scans for the diagnosis of isolated mandibular fractures is uncommon and may be cost-prohibitive. In our experience, the use of CT scans is reserved for cases involving complex (comminuted, avulsive, etc.) mandibular injuries or concomitant midfacial or orbital injuries. In some cases where a condylar fracture is suspected, the CT will allow for detailed three-dimensional imaging. Another useful application of the CT scan is in clinical situations (cervical spine injury, head injury) where the patient is not able to submit to routine radiographic positioning and techniques. Very young patients with limited cooperation may also be candidates for CT scan evaluation, but will often require sedation during the procedure. Magnetic resonance imaging (MRI) is of very limited value in evaluating bony injuries. It may be helpful to delineate injuries to the intracapsular structures of the TMJ, associated soft tissues or in cases of condylar displacement into the middle cranial fossa. Ultrasound has occasionally been used to determine condylar position after fractures.

4. Closed versus open treatment of mandibular fractures

Mandibular fractures have been successfully treated by closed-reduction methods for hundreds of years. Maxillomandibular fixation (MMF) is used to immobilize the fractured segments and allow osseous healing. When considering between open versus closed reduction of mandibular fractures the advantages should be weighed against the disadvantages. Considerations include the site and characteristics of the fracture and the morbidities of the treatment. Unwanted results including bony ankylosis or decreased mouth opening can be prevented by early mobilization of the mandible. Early mobilization helps to prevent possible ankylosis especially in patients with intracapsular fractures of the condyle. It is preferred to avoid maxillomandibular fixation when fractures involve the temporomandibular joint (TMJ) because postoperative physiotherapy can be started much earlier.

Advantages of closed reduction include simplicity, decreased operative time, and avoidance of damage to adjacent structures. Disadvantages of maxillomandibular fixation include inability to directly visualize the reduced fracture, need to keep the patient on a liquid diet, and difficulties with speech and respiration. The traditional length of immobilization of fractures when treated by closed reduction has been 6 weeks. Juniper and Awty found that 80% of mandibular fractures treated with open or closed reduction and maxillomandibular fixation had clinical union in 4 weeks [18]. They were able to show a correlation between the age of the patient and the predictability of early fracture union. Armaratunga found that 75% of mandible fractures had achieved clinical union by 4 weeks. Fractures in children healed in 2 weeks whereas a significant number of fractures in older patients took 8 weeks to achieve clinical union [19]. Although maxillomandibular fixation has long been considered a benign procedure it can be associated with significant problems. An excellent review of the deleterious effects of mandibular immobilization on the masticatory system is provided by Ellis [20]. Closed reduction of mandibular fractures can adversely affect bone, muscles, synovial joints, and periarticular connective tissues. The effects of immobilization on bone have been recognized in the orthopedic literature for many years as "disuse osteoporosis". Cortical and trabecular thinning, vascular distention, and increased osteoclastic activity have been described following joint immobilization [21]. Changes involving the musculature include not only muscle atrophy but also changes in muscle length and function.

5. Rigid fixation

Rigid fixation in the mandible refers to a form of treatment that consists of applying fixation to adequately reduce the fracture and also permit active use of the mandible during the healing process. The four AO/ASIF principles are

1. anatomical reduction
2. functionally stable fixation
3. atraumatic surgical technique

4.   immediate active function.

Although many osteosynthesis systems are currently available to treat mandibular fractures, the principles of plate application are similar. An overview of the various types follows.

5.1. Compression plates

Compression plates cause compression at the fracture site making primary bone healing more likely. These plates can be bent in only two dimensions because of their design and if they are not contoured properly they are unable to produce compression. It is important to avoid compressing oblique fractures. They also require bicortical screw engagement to produce even compression along the fracture line. This necessitates their placement at the inferior border to eliminate damage to the inferior alveolar neurovascular structures or the roots of the teeth. A higher incidence of complications has been noted in fractures treated with compression plates [22]. Because of the relatively small cross section of bone surface in some fractures, interfragmentary compression is often not possible. At our centre, surgeons prefer noncompression plates for treating mandibular fractures.

5.2. Reconstruction plates

Reconstruction plates are recommended for comminuted fractures and also for bridging continuity gaps. These plates are rigid and have corresponding screws with a diameter of 2.3–3.0 mm. Reconstruction plates can be adapted to the underlying bone and contoured in three dimensions. [Figure 3]

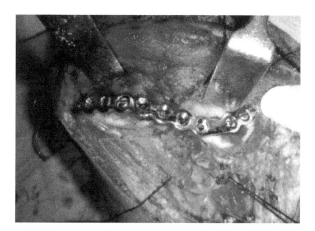

Figure 3. ORIF of a comminuted fracture using a Reconstruction Plate.

A problem that may be associated with conventional reconstruction plates is loosening of the screws during the healing process leading to instability of the fracture.

5.3. Locking reconstruction plates

In 1987 Raveh et al. introduced the titanium hollow-screw osteointegrated reconstruction plate (THORP) [23]. This system achieves stability between the screw and plate by insertion of an expansion screw into the head of the bone screw. This causes expansion of the screw flanges and locks them against the wall of the hole in the bone plate. Later Herford and Ellis described the use of locking reconstruction bone plate/screw system for mandibular surgery [24]. This system simplified the locking mechanism between the plate and the screw (Locking Reconstruction Plate, Synthes Maxillofacial, Paoli, PA) by engaging the threads of the head of the screw with the threads in the reconstruction plate, thus eliminating the need for expansion screws. Locking plate/screw systems offer advantages over conventional reconstruction plates. These plates function as internal fixators by achieving stability by locking the screw to the plate and allow greater stability as compared to conventional plates [25]. Fewer screws are required to maintain stability. The most significant advantage of this type of system is that it becomes unnecessary for the plate to intimately contact the underlying bone in all areas. As the screws are tightened they will not draw the plate and underlying bone toward each other.

5.4. Lag screw fixation

Lag screws can provide osteosynthesis of mandibular fractures [26,27]. They work well in oblique fractures and require a minimum of two screws. The lag screw engages the opposite cortex while fitting passively in the cortex of the outer bone segment. This can be accomplished by using a true lag screw or by overdrilling the proximal cortex. This causes compression of the osseous segments and provides the greatest rigidity of all fixation techniques. The proximal cortex should be countersunk to distribute the compressive forces over a broader area and avoid microfractures. The anatomy of the symphyseal region of the mandible lends itself to use of lag screws in a different technique. The lag screws can be placed through the opposing cortices between the mental foramen and inferior to the teeth. Fractures should not be oblique with this technique because it may cause the fractures to override each other.

5.5. Miniplates

Miniplates typically refer to small plates with a screw diameter of 2.0 mm. These plates have been shown to be effective in treating mandibular fractures. Typically a superior and inferior plate is required for adequate fixation. An exception to this is in the mandibular angle region where a superior border plate placed at the point of maximal tension is sufficient [Figure 4].

An advantage of these plates is that they are stable enough to obviate the need for maxillomandibular fixation and have a very low profile. They are less likely to be palpable, which reduces the need for subsequent plate removal. Typically screws are placed monocortically but may be placed bicortically when positioned along the inferior border of the mandible. A minimum of two screws should be placed in each osseous segment. Smaller incisions and less soft-tissue reflections are required with these plates when compared to larger plates and they can be placed from an intraoral approach, thus eliminating an external scar. Because these plates are less rigid than reconstruction plates, their use in treating comminuted fractures should be avoided. [28] A study at our centre evaluated the efficacy of 2.0-mm locking miniplate system versus 2.0-mm nonlocking miniplate system for mandibular fracture and concluded that both miniplate system present similar short-term complication rates. [29]

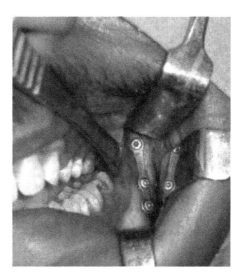

Figure 4. ORIF of an angle fracture using a single miniplate at the superior border.

5.6. Microminiplates

Microminiplates usually refer to small malleable plates with a screw diameter of 1.0–1.5 mm. Their use for mandibular surgery is limited because of their inability to provide rigid fixation and because they have a tendency for plate fracture during the healing process [30]. These plates can work well in the midface where the muscular forces are much less than those acting on the mandible. A recent study found a 30.4% complication rate when 1.3-mm microminiplates were used to provide osteosynthesis for mandibular fractures [31].

5.7. Bioresorbable plates

Bioresorbable plates are manufactured from varying amounts of materials including poly-dioxanone (PDS), polyglycolic acid, and polylactic acid. It has been shown that the breakage of a poly-L-lactic acid (PLLA) plate occurred at 50% of the yield strength required to break a miniplate [32]. Complications associated with these plates include inflammation and for-eign-body-type reactions. Laughlin et al. showed in their study that resorbable plates are equal to the performance of titanium 2-mm plates, regarding healing of the fracture with bone union and restoration of function. [33] We are also using resorbable plates for routine treatment of mandibular fractures. [Figure 5]

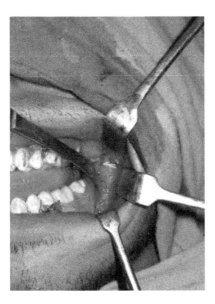

Figure 5. ORIF using a resorbable plate at the angle region.

The common complication which we encountered during their use was screw head fracture during tightening. Consideration may be given for use in pediatric patients with the understanding of the possible complications.

5.8. Three-dimensional miniplates

These miniplates are based on the principle that when a geometrically closed quadrangular plate is secured with bone screws, it creates stability in three dimensions. The smallest structural component of a 3-D-plate is an open cube or a square stone. [Figure 6]

Clinical results and biomechanical investigations in a study have shown a good stability of the 3-D-plates in the osteosynthesis of mandibular fractures without major complications. The thin 1.0 mm connecting arms of the plate allow easy adaptation to the bone without distortion. The free areas between the arms permit good blood supply to the bone. [34]. A study conducted at our center showed that there is no major difference in terms of treatment outcome between conventional and 3-Dimensional Miniplates, and both are equally effective in managing mandibular fracture. [35] We believe 3- D miniplates provide good stability and operative time is less because of simultaneous stabilization at both superior and inferior borders.

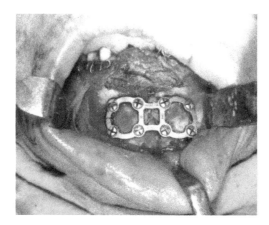

Figure 6. ORIF using a 3-Dimensional plate at symphysis fracture site.

6. General principles

6.1. Surgical technique

Intermaxillary fixation is placed prior to reducing a fracture. This allows for use of the occlusion to aid in anatomical reduction of the fracture. Use of full-arch bars combined with maxillomandibular fixation is the preferred method. The arch bars provide a way to maintain the occlusion postoperatively with elastic bands as needed during physiotherapy. The arch bars are usually removed after 4 weeks postoperatively.

The surgical approach depends on the site of the fracture. Either a transoral, vestibular, or transfacial approach may be performed. A facial approach provides excellent access but also produces a facial scar and adds the risk of damage to the facial nerve. Most fractures, excluding those of the condyle, can easily be approached through a transoral incision. A subperiosteal dissection with a periosteal elevator provides adequate access for reduction of the fracture and placement of fixation. Attention should be given to avoiding damage to the mental nerve, which exists the mental foramen near the apices of the premolar teeth. If additional exposure is needed, the nerve can be released by gently scoring the periosteum surrounding the nerve. Bone-reducing forceps are often helpful in reducing the fracture while adapting the bone plate. This also provides interfragmentary compression, making primary bone healing more likely. The smallest bone plate that will provide adequate stability under functional loads during the healing period is chosen. A minimum of two screws on either side of the fracture is required. Larger, more rigid plates are required to treat comminuted fractures or continuity defects [24]. The intermaxillary fixation that aided reduction of the fractures during plating is removed after the fixation is applied. A soft diet is recommended for at least 3 weeks after miniplate fixation. It is important during the postoperative period to regain preinjury function, including maximal mouth opening, with active physiotherapy.

6.1.1. Teeth in the line of fracture

Most teeth in the line of fracture can be saved if appropriate antibiotic therapy and fixation techniques are used. Indications for removal of teeth in the line of fracture include grossly mobile teeth, partly erupted third molars with pericoronitis, teeth that prevent reduction of the fractures, fractured tooth roots, entire exposed root surfaces, or an excessive delay from the time of fracture to treatment. [36,37]

6.1.2. Antibiotics and mandible fractures

Zallen and Curry showed that mandibular fractures were associated with a 50% infection rate when patients did not receive antibiotic therapy. The infection rate was reduced to 6% for those patients who received antibiotics [38].

7. Treatment of specific fractures

7.1. Symphysis fractures

The optimal management of symphyseal and parasymphyseal fractures continue to evolve. Fractures in this area of the mandible predispose the patients to malocclusion and widening of the face if not properly treated. Arch bars and MMF are necessary to establish the pre-morbid relationship of the mandibular and maxillary teeth. However, care must be taken to avoid overtightening the MMF, which can cause flaring of the mandibular angles. The most common approach to the symphysis and parasymphysis is the transoral gingivolabial and gingivobuccal incision. With larger, comminuted fractures, an external approach may be necessary to accurately and rigidly fixate the mandible. Simple symphysis fractures can be treated with two miniplates. Because of the torsional forces generated during function, a single miniplate is insufficient to predictably maintain rigid fixation during healing [39]. One miniplate is placed at the inferior border and a second plate is placed superiorly. The superior plate is secured with a minimum of two monocortical screws in each segment whereas bicortical screws can be used on the inferior plate. Care should be taken to avoid damage to tooth roots while fixing the superior plate. These plates were placed in accordance to Champy's line of osteosynthesis. [Figure 7]

Several authors have shown that miniplate fixation along these lines is a very effective way to fixate these fractures. [40]

More rigid fixation should be considered for comminuted fractures. It is important to avoid "flaring" of the ramus in patients with a symphysis fracture and especially when combined with condyle fractures. This will be seen clinically as a dental crossbite of the posterior occlusion and also fullness of the mandibular angle region. This can be avoided by applying pressure at the angle region during fixation, overbending the plate(s), and directly visualizing the lingual aspect of the reduced fracture.

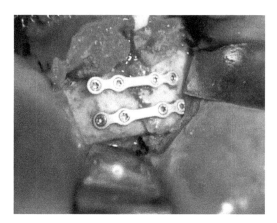

Figure 7. ORIF of symphysis fracture using two miniplates; one at the superior border and other at the inferior border along Champy's line of osteosynthesis.

Lag screw fixation is other useful technique in the symphysis and parasymphysis region [41]. When the lag screws are applied, it is imperative to reduce the lingual border of the fracture and re-establish the appropriate intergonial distance by squeezing the mandibular angles together. While holding the reduction, the lag screws may be applied. For optimal strength, two lag screws are placed. Several authors have suggested that a single strong plate with an arch bar is adequate in managing symphyseal fractures. We are also using single strong plates at inferior border along with arch bar as a tension band in our cases. No major complications have been noted in any of our patients.

7.1.1. Mandibular body fractures

Simple fractures involving the body of the mandible can be effectively treated with one miniplate along the Champy line of osteosynthesis. [Figure 8]

Care should be taken during the dissection to avoid damaging the mental nerve, which supplies sensation to the lower lip. If further reflection is necessary, the periosteum can be scored to release the nerve and allow improved visualization. Often a bone-reducing clamp can be applied prior to plate placement to aid in reduction of the fracture.

7.1.2. Angle fractures

The angle region of the mandible is one of the most common sites of fracture. Often trauma to the lateral mandible will cause a fracture at the angle and also involve the contralateral mandible. Many reasons for the greater proportion of fractures to this site have been cited. These include the presence of impacted third molars, a thinner cross-sectional area in this region, and also the biomechanical lever arm in this area. A recent study looked at the incidence of fractures when teeth were involved. They found a significantly increased incidence of fractures involving the mandibular angle when there was an associated impacted third molar [42]. The angle region is a weak point, because the bone anterior and posterior (body and ramus, respectively) are thicker than the bone in the angle region [43]. These fractures are associated with the highest rate of complications [18]. The angle fracture can be further complicated by distraction and rotation by opposing forces of the elevator muscles (masseter, medial and lateral pterygoid, temporalis) and the depressor muscles (geniohyoid, genioglossus, mylohyoid, digastrics).

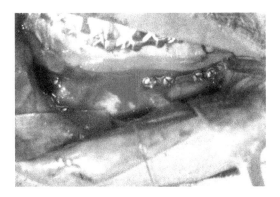

Figure 8. ORIF of a mandibular body fracture with a single miniplate between root apices and inferior alveolar canal along Champy's line of osteosynthesis.

Many techniques for treating mandibular angle fractures have been described. Because no teeth are present in the posterior (proximal) segment, arch bars cannot be used to stabilize the segments and there is no control over the proximal segment. Closed-reduction techniques are often associated with rotation of the ramus. With the introduction of plate-and-screw osteosynthesis many surgical methods have been described. Those who advocate large bone plates are attempting to eliminate interfragment mobility and thus allow for primary bone union [23,44]. Others have questioned the need for absolute rigidity for treatment of angle fractures In 1973, Michelet et al. described the use of small, malleable bone plates for treatment of angle fractures [13]. This led to a change from the previous belief that rigid fixation was necessary for bone healing. Later, Champy et al. validated the technique by performing several clinical investigations [14]. They determined the most stable location where bone plates should be placed based on the "ideal lines of osteosynthesis". The "Champy technique" involves placing a small bone plate along the superior border and using monocortical screws to secure the plate and avoid damage to the adjacent teeth or inferior alveolar neurovascular bundle. Absolute immobilization is not provided with this form of treatment (semirigid fixation). Clinical studies have shown that the amount of stability of the fractures is significant enough to eliminate the need for maxillomandibular fixation [45].

The superior border plate neutralizes distraction forces (tension) on the mandible while preserving the self-compressive forces that occur during function.

A prospective study looked at eight methods for treating mandibular angle fractures [45]:

1. closed reduction;

2. extraoral ORIF with a large reconstruction plate;

3. intraoral ORIF using a single lag screw;

4. intraoral ORIF using two 2.0-mm minidynamic compression plates;

5. intraoral ORIF using two 2.4-mm mandibular compression plate;

6. intraoral ORIF using two noncompression miniplates;

7. intraoral ORIF using a single noncompression miniplate; and

8. intraoral ORIF using a single malleable noncompression miniplate.

The results revealed that extraoral ORIF with a reconstruction plate and intraoral ORIF using a single miniplate are associated with the fewest complications (7.5% and 2.5%, respectively). This finding is interesting because the single miniplate is less rigid than the other forms of fixation, yet it is associated with the fewest complications. A possible explanation is that less extensive dissection is required and more of the blood supply is maintained.

We are also using intraoral ORIF using a single miniplate along the Champy's ideal line of osteosynthesis for angle fractures. [Figure 9]

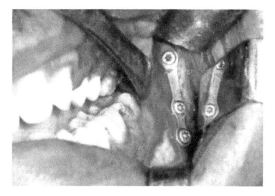

Figure 9. Intraoral ORIF using a single miniplate along the Champy's ideal line of osteosynthesis for angle fractures.

The main problem we encountered is the inability to achieve anatomic reduction in cases of severely displaced angle fractures through intraoral approach. A study conducted at our centre evaluated the efficacy of using a single miniplate at the inferior border in the management of a displaced angle fracture through extraoral approach. [Figure 10-12]

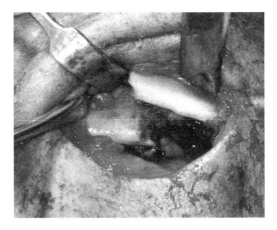

Figure 10. Intraoperative view showing displaced angle fracture exposed through extraoral approach.

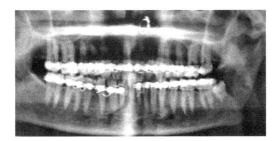

Figure 11. Panoramic Tomogram showing displaced left angle fracture.

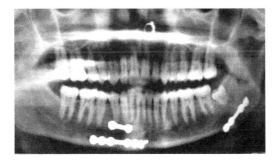

Figure 12. Panoramic Tomogram showing anatomically reduced angle fracture and fixation with a single miniplate at inferior border.

The study concluded that outcomes are acceptable in patients but a multicenter study with an appropriate comparison group is required to substantiate a more generalizable conclusion of efficacy of this single miniplate at inferior border. [46]

7.1.3. Condyle fractures

Fractures of the condyle can involve the head (intracapsular), neck, or subcondylar region. The head of the condyle may be dislocated outside of the fossa. The most common direction of displacement is in an anteromedial direction because of the pull from the lateral pterygoid muscle, which inserts on the anterior portion of the head of the condyle. No other type of mandibular fracture is associated with as much controversy regarding treatment as those involving the condyle. Factors considered in deciding whether to treat a condyle fracture open or closed include the fracture level, amount of displacement, adequacy of the occlusion, and whether the patient can tolerate maxillomandibular fixation. Those who advocate open treatment cite advantages including early mobilization of the mandible, better occlusal results, better function, maintenance of posterior ramal height, and avoidance of facial asymmetries [47]. The ramal height shortening can be assessed on panoramic radiograph [Figure 13] and can be restored by open treatment of condylar fractures. [Figure 14]

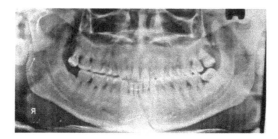

Figure 13. Panoramic Tomogram showing displaced right subcondylar fracture and left parasymphysis fracture. Note that there is loss of ramal height on the right side.

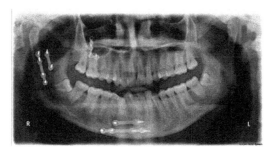

Figure 14. Panoramic Tomogram of fixation of subcondylar fracture using two miniplates; the vertical ramal height is restored by ORIF of subcondylar fracture.

Others prefer closed reduction mainly because of the possible complications associated with open reduction including damage to branches of the facial nerve and a cutaneous scar. Recently endoscopic subcondylar fracture repair has been described with encouraging results [48]. Nonsurgical management (closed reduction) includes MMF with elastics for a variable period followed by guiding elastics so as to maintain the occlusion while allowing jaw physiotherapy during healing. Measurable criteria should be assessed whether treating by closed or open methods. These should include pain-free movement, mouth-opening, jaw movement in all excursions, preinjury occlusion, radiographic assessment of deviation of the fractured fragment and shortening of the ascending ramus [49]. Zide and Kent described the absolute and relative indications for open reduction of condyle fractures [50]. Absolute indications include

1. displacement of the condylar head into the middle cranial fossa;

2. impossibility of obtaining adequate occlusion by closed reduction;

3. lateral extracapsular displacement of the condyle; and

4. invasion by a foreign body (e.g.gunshot wound)

Relative indications include

1. bilateral condyle fractures in an edentulous patient;

2. unilateral or bilateral condyle fractures when splinting is not recommended for medical reasons;

3. bilateral condyle fractures associated with comminuted midface fractures; and

4. bilateral condyle fractures and associated gnathological problems (e.g. lack of posterior occlusal support).

The degree of displacement of the condylar fracture has been used in deciding between open or closed treatment. Mikkonen et al. and Klotch and Lundy recommended open reduction if the condylar displacement was greater than 45 degrees in a sagittal or coronal plane and Widmark et al. recommended opening such fractures if the displacement was greater than 30 degrees [51-53]. The author proposed a new classification of subcondylar fractures of the mandible based on ramal height shortening and degree of fracture angulation. [54] The classification is as follows:

8. Fracture classification

On the basis of Towne's and panoramic radiograph, the fractures are categorized into 3 classes:

1. 1Class 1 (minimally displaced)—fracture with ramal height shortening; < 2 mm and/or degree of fracture displacement; <10°.

2. Class 2 (moderately displaced)—fracture with ramal height shortening; 2 to 15 mm and/or degree of fracture displacement; 10 to 35°

3. Class 3 (severely displaced)—fracture with ramal height shortening; >15 mm and/or degree of fracture displacement; >35°.

This new classification based on ramal height shortening and degree of fracture displacement can better guide clinical treatment. Class 1 fractures should be treated by closed method, while open reduction is recommended in Class 2 and Class 3 cases.

Intracapsular fractures involving the condylar head are difficult to treat and most recommend close treatment of these fractures to avoid damage to adjacent structures. Fractures involving the condylar neck and subcondylar region can be approached with less morbidity. Many surgical approaches have been described with the most common being the retromandibular, submandibular, and preauricular approaches [55]. A nerve stimulator can be helpful in identifying branches of the facial nerve during the dissection. A prospective study compared the effect on facial symmetry after either closed or open treatment of mandibular condylar process fractures [56]. It was found that treatment by closed methods led to asymmetries characterized by shortening of the face on the side of the injury. The loss of posterior height on the side of fracture is an adaptation that helps re-establish a new temporomandibular articulation. Loss of facial height on the affected side can lead to compensatory canting of the occlusal plane. Treatment of condylar process fractures should be individualized. Many factors, including the patient's own preference, should be considered. Whether surgical or nonsurgical treatment is chosen, we recommend early mobilization during the healing process.

8.1. Pediatric fractures

The management of pediatric fractures is complicated by the presence of deciduous teeth and the growing mandible. Children tend to be less tolerant of MMF. An acrylic splint can be helpful in managing mandibular fractures in children. [Figure 15]

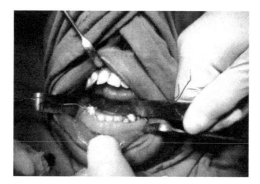

Figure 15. Intraoperative view of use of acrylic splint in managing mandibular fractures in children.

This can be used without MMF to allow early postoperative physiotherapy to avoid ankylosis and/or growth disturbances, which are more common in pediatric patients [57].

Condylar process fractures in children younger than age 12 should be treated by closed methods in most instances. Damage to the condylar growth center can result in delayed growth and in facial asymmetry. Dalhlstrom et al. showed good restitution of the TMJ and no growth disturbances in 14 children, 5 years after nonsurgical treatment of their fractures [58].

Early animal studies showed that there was little sacrifice of mandibular growth and symmetry with induced condyle fractures when treated with closed reduction. Boyne compared three methods of fracture treatment in Rhesus monkeys and found no difference between those treated with internal fixation (wire), MMF, or no treatment [59].

8.2. Edentulous fractures

Fractures of the edentulous mandible most commonly involve the body region. Changes that occur with age include decreased osteogenesis, mandibular atrophy, and reduced blood supply. With age the inferior alveolar artery contributes less and less to perfusion of the mandible [60]. The lack of teeth makes it difficult to adequately reduce the fracture because MMF cannot be used to help reduce the bony fragments. It is important to define more carefully 'edentulous' mandibles, since the literature shows that only those severely atrophic mandibles with a bone height less than 10 mm stand out as a 'difficult' or special problem. Above these heights, normal miniplate fixation may be effective.

These fractures can be treated by either open or closed reduction methods. Closed techniques often involve wiring a mandibular prosthesis in place with circumandibular wires to stabilize the fracture. The second Chalmers J. Lyons Academy Study of fractures of the edentulous mandible reviewed 167 fractures in 104 edentulous mandibles. Fifteen percent of the patients developed a delayed fibrous union and 26% treated by closed reduction techniques had problems with union. The fewest complications occurred with the patients who received transfacial open reduction and internal fixation [61].

In addition to adequate reduction and stabilization of the fractured segments, the successful management of fractures involving the edentulous mandible requires that consideration be given to the amount of bone present. When the mandible is severely atrophic, it is possible that healing will not occur even if open reduction and internal fixation principles are properly applied. In some circumstances, treatment consists of simultaneous bone graft reconstruction at the time of fracture repair. This is also appropriate treatment for patients presenting with non-union of an edentulous fracture. In most cases plans for definitive prosthetic reconstruction are delayed until full healing of the bony site has occurred. Some authors, however, do advocate early reconstruction with bone grafting and osseo-integrated implants. [62]

Treatment methods for edentulous mandible fractures

- Closed reduction with the use of prosthetics (existing dentures or Gunning splints

- External fixation

- Wire fixation

- Open reduction with internal fixation:

1. reconstruction plates (2.3-2.7 mm diameter screws)

2. mandible fixation plates (2.0-2.4 mm diameter screws):

    - dynamic compression plates

    - plates at both inferior and superior borders of the fracture

3. bone grafting and miniplate fixation

8.3. Infected fractures

Infected mandibular fractures resulting from a delay in treatment can present certain challenges. Treatment by MMF, external fixation, and rigid internal fixation has been recommended. The goals of treating mandibular fractures that are complicated by an infection include resolution of the infection and achievement of bony union. Rigid internal fixation can predictably be used for treatment of infected mandibular fractures [63]. Fracture union and resolution can be attained with fixation. Even if the infection is prolonged, the fracture can heal as long as rigidity of the fracture is maintained. The plate can be removed after the bony union is achieved. Alternatively, if it is noted that plate or screw loosening has occurred and rigidity between the osseous segments is lacking, a nonunion is likely. The patient should be treated to regain rigidity and eliminate any loose hardware.

9. Complications

Complications following mandible fracture repair may be the result of the severity of the original injury, the surgical treatment or patient non-compliance with the postoperative regimen. Problems related to mandibular fractures present unique challenges to even the most experienced surgeon. The consequences of complications may include problems in anatomic form (cosmetic deformity) or residual functional disturbances. Complication rates have improved since the early days of wire fixation, but even the most sound fixation techniques can yield undesirable results. Probably no other specific area of oral and maxillofacial surgery has been studied in more detail than the mandible fracture. Despite this fact, little prospective evidence is available regarding the outcomes of the various treatment modalities. Retrospective studies offer some evidence that certain techniques have independently done better than others, but better prospective studies are needed to further evaluate and compare these techniques.

9.1. Malocclusion and malunion

Improper alignment of the fracture fragments results in facial asymmetry and malocclusion. Malunions occur in 0–4.2% of fractures. Malunions result from improper reduction, insufficient immobilization, poor patient compliance, and the improper use of rigid internal fixation [64]. Residual arch form deformity following the surgical repair of a mandibular fracture is often the result of inadequate reduction. Failure to re-establish the anatomic configuration of the arch form result in occlusal prematurities and misalignment which will compromise masticatory function. Clinicians treating mandibular fractures need to be familiar with dental anatomy and occlusion in order to balance the functional forces appropriately. Preoperative study models (with or without model surgery) and splint fabrication may aid in fracture reduction in some cases. Poor apposition of fracture segments may results from a delay in or an absence of treatment, inadequate treatment, inability to align segments secondary to the presence of a foreign body or loss of bony landmarks. Malaligned fracture segments noted early in the postoperative course may be corrected by returning to the operating room for removal of the hardware and repeat reduction with internal fixation. When the discrepancies are not caught early, the fracture segments will go on to heal in the improper anatomic position (malunion). Significant malunions of the mandible will produce asymmetry and/or functional disturbances and can only be resolved through carefully planned osteotomies for reconstruction of the mandibular arch form. The most common cause of failure of fracture healing (non-union) is residual mobility across the fracture site. Movement of the bone ends will disrupt the fibrovascular structures, decrease the recruitment of osteoprogenitor cells and allow for fibrous tissue ingrowth instead of bony healing. Other contributors to fracture non-union include impaired healing capacity secondary to illness, tobacco use and infection. Non-union of mandibular fractures requires reoperation to excise any fibrous tissue within the fracture gap in combination with application of bone fixation. In some instances, there may be loss of bone, producing a continuity defect which will require bone graft reconstruction. Treatment strategies vary from patient to patient and with each surgeon's experience in using different techniques.

Comprehensive management of malocclusion and malunion requires a full orthognathic workup. Standard osteotomies are performed at a different site from the malunion for restoration of preinjury occlusion. In general, treatment involves osteotomies at the healed fracture sites if they are within the dental arch, whereas fractures proximal to the dental arch are treated with ramus procedures.

9.2. Infection

Infection, the most common complication of mandibular fractures, is reported in 0.4–32% of all cases [64]. The potential for infection is always a consideration when treating fractures of the mandible, especially when there is communication with the oral cavity (e.g. compound fracture). Other risk indicators for increased chance of infection include active substance abuse and non-compliance with postoperative regimens [65] A significant delay in treatment has also been associated with an increase in infection rates. [66] Other factors include mobility of the segments across the fracture site or loosening of screws securing the plate. Poor plate adaptation, inadequate cooling during drilling, or placing the screw in the fracture line itself can lead to increased chance of infection developing. Leaving a tooth in the line of fracture can also lead to an increased incidence of complications. Of the facial bones, the mandible is the most frequently infected region following surgical intervention for traumatic injury. This is likely due to instability of the segments from muscular actions on the proximal and distal segments and the density of the bone. Manifestations of infection include cellulitis, abscess formation, fistula, osteomyelitis and rarely necrotizing fasciitis. [Figure 16]

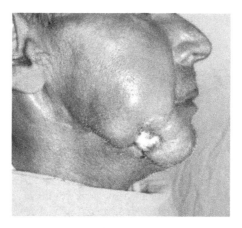

Figure 16. Patient with non-union of body fracture of edentulous mandible; exposed necrotic bone with pus discharge can be noticed.

Management begins with clinical examination and plain radiographic studies to assess the status of the fractured segments and the hardware. The use of CT and MRI is appropriate when there is concern that the infection involves the surrounding soft tissues of the neck. Specimens for bacterial culture and sensitivity studies should be done as early as possible in the patient's clinical course.

Infections involving rigid fixation of mandibular fractures may not necessitate plate removal (minor) or may be major and require plate removal (loose hardware). Treatment of the infection requires antibiotics and determination of the stability of the fracture. The fracture site can heal and develop union in the face of infection as long as there is rigidity across the fracture site.

9.3. Delayed union and nonunion

Delayed union is failure of fracture union by 2 months. Infection, mobility, systemic disease, advanced age, and mandibular atrophy are contributing factors [64]. Delayed union by definition means that the fracture will eventually heal without further surgery. Rigid internal fixation carries a lower incidence of delayed union compared to nonrigid fixation: 0–2.8% versus 1–4.4% [64].

Nonunion is the failure of a fracture to unite owing to arrested healing and requiring additional treatment to achieve fracture union. Mobility is the major cause of nonunion. More than 33% of nonunions involve infection [64]. Large bony gaps, traumatized devitalized tissue, older age, intervening soft tissue, and systemic disease all can contribute to nonunion. Mobility at the fracture site is manifested in nonunions. Debridement of the fracture fragments, bone grafting, usually from the iliac crest, and rigid fixation with internal or external fixation usually achieves fracture union. [Figure 17]

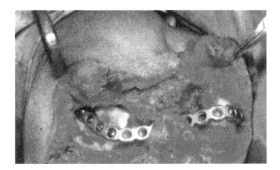

Figure 17. Placement of a Locking Reconstuction Plate for treatment of a mandibular non-union site.

9.4. Nerve injury

Sensory nerve injury, particularly of the inferior alveolar and mental nerves, commonly occurs with mandibular fractures [67]. In 11–59% of displaced mandibular fractures there is sensory nerve injury at diagnosis [68,69]. Most injuries are neuropraxias secondary to stretching or compression and resolve spontaneously. Causes of inferior alveolar or mental nerve injury are displaced fractures, delay in treatment, and improper use of drill or screws. Facial nerve dysfunction infrequently results from mandibular trauma. Damage to the facial nerve in temporal bone fractures can lead to paralysis. Retrograde edema distal to the geniculate ganglion can cause temporary facial nerve loss after condylar fractures. Condylar dislocations can cause facial nerve injury distal to the stylomastoid foramen. Injury to the facial nerve branches usually takes place iatrogenically during surgical treatment, though lateral displacement of the condyle can cause facial nerve injury [69]. The marginal mandibular branch is the one usually injured. The surgical anatomy of this branch has been well described by Dingman and Grabb [70], and meticulous dissection under the platysma in the region of the facial artery with identification of the branches of the marginal mandibular nerve can prevent injury to this nerve [71]. The design of the preauricular incision in the approach to the condyle can be accomplished by observing the landmark work of Al-Kayat and Bramley [72].

Patients with a paresthesia following a mandibular fracture should be observed during the postoperative period and the level of neurosensory return (subjective) is documented. In cases where patients report no improvement in their level of sensation after 6-8 weeks, the clinician may consider obtaining baseline nerve function data using objective testing. Objective neurosensory testing before 6 weeks may be of limited value because it is difficult to discern a Sunderland Class I injury (excellent prognosis without surgery) from a Sunderland Class V injury (poor prognosis without surgery) that early in the postoperative course. In the case of Sunderland Class IV and V injuries (equivalent to axonotmesis and neurotmesis) surgical repair is considered between 3 and 6 months [73]. Immediate management of inferior alveolar nerve injury at the time of mandibular fracture repair has been advocated in situations where there is displacement at the fracture site and anesthesia [74]. Although a more aggressive approach may have merit, it would be limited to situations where there is an observed transection of the nerve. Immediate decompression and exploration are not necessary in less severe nerve injuries (Sunderland Class I, II, III) and surgical maneuvers used to expose the nerve trunk (decortication) may compromise subsequent fracture healing

Author details

Amrish Bhagol[1*], Virendra Singh[1] and Ruchi Singhal[2]

*Address all correspondence to: bhagol.amrish@gmail.com

1 Department of Oral and Maxillofacial Surgery, Post Graduate Institute of Dental Sciences, Pt. B.D. Sharma University of Health Sciences, Rohtak, Haryana, India

2 Department of Pedodontic and Preventive Dentistry, Post Graduate Institute of Dental Sciences, Pt. B.D. Sharma University of Health Sciences, Rohtak, HaryanaIndia,

References

[1] The Edwin Smith Surgical Papyrus (trans. Breasted JH) University of Chicago Press, Chicago 1930

[2] Lipton JS. Oral surgery in ancient Egypt as reflected in the Edwin Smith Papyrus. Bulletin of the History of Dentistry 1982; 30: 108

[3] Hippocrates. Oeuvres completes (English trans. Withington ET) Cambridge, MA 1928

[4] Salicetti G. Cyrurgia 1275

[5] Prevost N. Translation of Salicetti's Cyrurgia. Lyons, France 1492

[6] Gilmer TL. A case of fracture of the lower jaw with remarks on the treatment. Archives of Dentistry 1887; 4: 388

[7] Ivy RH. Fracture of condyloid process of the mandible. Annals of Surgery 1915; 61: 502

[8] Buck G. Fracture of the lower jaw with replacement and interlocking of the fragments. Annalist NY 1846; 1:245.

[9] Dorrance GM, Bransfield JW. The History of Treatment of Fractured Jaws, vols 1 and 2. Washington, DC, 1941.

[10] Gilmer TL. Fractures of the inferior maxilla. Ohio State J Dent Sci 1881-1882;1: 309;2:14,57, 112.

[11] Luhr HG: Zur Stabilen osteosynthese bei Unterkeiferfrakturen. Dtsch Zahnarztl Z 1968;23: 754.

[12] Spiessl B. New concepts in maxillofacial bone surgery. Springer-Verlag, Berlin 1976

[13] Michelet FX, Deymes J. Dessus B. Osteosynthesis with miniaturized screwed plates in maxillofacial surgery. J Maxillofac Surg 1973; 1: 79.

[14] Champy M, Lodde JP, Schmitt R, et al. Mandibular osteosynthesis by miniature screwed plates via a buccal approach. J Maxillofac Surg 1978;6: 14.

[15] Suuronen R. Biodegradable fracture fixation devices in maxillofacial surgery. International Journal of Oral and Maxillofacial Surgery 1993;22: 50

[16] Eppley BL, Prevel CD, Sarver D. Resorbable bone fixation: its potential role in craniomaxillofacial trauma. Journal of Craniomaxillofacial Trauma 1996;2: 56

[17] Chayra GA, Meador LR, Laskin OM. Comparison of panoramic and standard radiographs for the diagnosis of mandibular fractures. Journal of Oral and Maxillofacial Surgery 1985;44; 677

[18] Juniper RP, Awty MD. The immobilization period for fractures of the mandibular body. J Oral Surg 1973; 36:157.

[19] Armaratunga NA de S. The relation of age to the Immobilization period required for healing of mandibular fractures. J Oral Maxillofac Surg 1987; 45:111.

[20] Ellis E. The effects of mandibular immobilization on the masticatory system: a review. Clin Plast Surg 1989; 16:133–146.

[21] Geiser M, Trueta J. Muscle action, bone rarefaction and bone formation: an experimental study. J Bone Joint Surg 1958; 40B:282–311.

[22] Iizuka T, Lindqvist C. Rigid internal fixation of fractures in the angular region of the mandible: an analysis of factors contributing to different complications. Plast Reconstr Surg 1993; 91:265–271

[23] Raveh J, Vuillemin T, Ladrach K, et al. Plate osteosynthesis of 367 mandibular fractures. J Craniomaxillofac Surg 1987; 15:244–253.

[24] Herford AS, Ellis E. Use of a locking reconstruction plate=screw system for mandibular surgery. J Oral Maxillofac Surg 1998; 56(11):1261–1265.

[25] Soderholm A-L, Lindqvist C, Skutnabb K, et al. Bridging of mandibular defects with two different reconstruction systems: an experimental study. J Oral Maxillofac Surg 1991; 49:1098.

[26] Niederdellman H, Shetty V. Solitary lag screw osteosynthesis in the treatment of fractures of the angle of the mandible: a retrospective study. Plast Reconstr Surg 1987; 80(1):68–74.

[27] Forrest CR. Application of minimal-access techniques in lag screw fixation of fractures of the anterior mandible. Plast Reconstr Surg 1999; 104:2127–2134.

[28] Edwards TJ, David DJ. A comparative study of miniplates used in the treatment of mandibullar fractures. Plast Reconstr Surg 1996; 97(6):1150–1157.

[29] Singh V, Kumar I, Bhagol A. Comparative evaluation of 2.0-mm locking plate system vs 2.0-mm nonlocking plate system for mandibular fracture: a prospective randomized study. Int J Oral Maxillofac Surg. 2011; 40(4):372-7.

[30] Potter J, Ellis E. Treatment of mandibular angle fractures with a malleable noncompression miniplate. J Oral Maxillofac Surg 1999; 57:288–292.

[31] Kim YK, Nam KW. Treatment of mandible fractures using low-profile titanium miniplates: preliminary study. Plast Reconstr Surg 2001; 108:38–43.

[32] Bos RRM, Boering G, Rozema FR, et al. Resorbable poly (L-lactide) plates and screws for the fixation of zygomatic fractures. J Oral Maxillofac Surg 1987; 45:751.

[33] Laughlin RM, Block MS, Wilk R, Malloy RB, Kent JN. Resorbable plates for the fixation of mandibular fractures: a prospective study. J Oral Maxillofac Surg. 2007 ;65(1): 89-96

[34] Farmand M. Experiences with the 3-D miniplate osteosynthesis in mandibular fractures. Fortschr Kiefer Gesichtschir. 1996; 41:85-7.

[35] Singh V, Puri P, Arya S, Malik S, Bhagol A. Conventional versus 3-Dimensional Miniplate in Management of Mandibular Fracture -A Prospective Randomized Study. Otolaryngol Head Neck Surg. May 2012 (Online Published)

[36] Neal DC, Wagner W, Alpert B. Morbidity associated with teeth in the line of mandibular fractures. J Oral Surg 1978; 36:859.

[37] Shetty V, Freymiller E. Teeth in the line of fracture: a review. J Oral Maxillofac Surg 1989; 47:1303.

[38] Zallen RD, Curry JT. A study of antibiotic usage in compound mandibular fractures. J Oral Surg 1975; 33:431.

[39] Champy M, Lodde JP, Schmitt R, et al.Mandibular osteosynthesis by miniature screwed bone plates via a buccal approach. J Oral Maxillofac Surg 1978; 6:14.

[40] Chritah A, Lazow SK, Berger J. Transoral 2.0-mm miniplate fixation of mandibular fractures plus 2 weeks maxillomandibular fixation: A prospective study. J Oral Maxillofac Surg 2002; 60:167-170.

[41] Ellis E 3rd. Lag screw fixation of mandibular fractures. J Craniomaxillofac Trauma 1997; 3: 16-26

[42] Fuselier JC, Ellis E, Dodson TB. Do mandibular third molars alter the risk of angle fractures? J Oral Maxillofac Surg 2002; 60(5):514–518.

[43] Shubert W, Kobienia BJ, Pollock RA. Cross-sectional area of the mandible. J Oral Maxillofac Surg 1997; 55:689–692.

[44] Becker R. Stable compression plate fixation of mandibular fractures. Br J Oral Surg 1974; 12:13–23.

[45] Ellis E III. Treatment methods for fractures of the mandibular angle. Int J Oral Maxillofac Surg 1999; 28(4):243–252.

[46] Singh V, Gupta M, Bhagol A. Is a Single Miniplate at the Inferior Border Adequate in the Management of an Angle Fracture of the Mandible? Otolaryngol Head Neck Surg. 2011;145(2):213-6.

[47] Ellis E, Throckmorton G. Facial symmetry after closed and open treatment of fractures of the mandibular condylar process. J Oral Maxillofac Surg 2000; 58(7):719–728.

[48] Martin M, Lee C. Endoscopic mandibular condyle fracture repair. Atlas Oral Maxillofac Surg Clin North Am. 2003;11(2):169-78.

[49] Singh V, Bhagol A, Goel M, Kumar I, Verma A. Outcomes of Open Versus Closed Treatment of Mandibular Subcondylar Fractures: A Prospective Randomized Study. J Oral Maxillofac Surg. 2010;68(6):1304-9

[50] Zide MF, Kent JN. Indications for open reduction of mandibular condyle fractures. J Oral Maxillofac Surg 1983; 41:89.

[51] Mikkonen P, Lindqvist C, Pihakari A, et al: Osteotomy–osteosynthesis in displaced condylar fractures. Int J Oral Maxillofac Surg 1989; 18:267.

[52] Klotch DW, Lundy LB. Condylar neck fractures of the mandible. Otolaryngol Clin North Am 1991; 24:181.

[53] Widmark G, Bagenholm T, Kahnberg KE, et al: Open reduction of subcondylar fractures. Int J Oral Maxillofac Surg 1996; 25:107.

[54] Bhagol A, Singh V, Kumar I, Verma A. Prospective Evaluation of a New Classification System for the Management of Mandibular Subcondylar Fractures.. J Oral Maxillofac Surg. 2010;68(6):1304-9

[55] Ellis E, Dean J. Rigid Fixation of mandibular condyle fractures. Oral Surg Oral Pathol 1993; 76:6.

[56] Ellis E, Throckmorton G, Palmieri C. Open treatment of condylar process fractures: assessment of adequacy of repositioning and maintenance of stability. J Oral Maxillo-fac Surg 2000; 58:27–34.

[57] Kaban LB, Mulliken MD, Murray JE. Facial fractures in children: an analysis of 122 fractures in 109 patients. Plast Reconstr Surg 1977; 59:15.

[58] Dahlstrom L, Kahnberg KE, Lindahl. 15 years follow-up on condylar fractures. Int J Oral Maxillofac Surg 1989; 18(1):18–23.

[59] Boyne PJ. Osseous repair and mandibular growth after subcondylar fractures. J Oral Surg 1967; 25(4):300–309.

[60] Bradley JC. Age changes in the vascular supply of the mandible. Br Dent J 1972; 132(4):142–144.

[61] Bruce RA, Ellis E III. The second Chalmers J Lyons Academy study of fractures of the edentulous mandible. J Oral Maxillofac Surg 1993; 51(8):904–911.

[62] Eyrich GK, Gratz Kw, Sailer HF. Surgical treatment ofthe edentulous mandible. Jour-nal of Oral and Maxillofacial Surgery 1997;55: 1081-1087

[63] Koury M, Ellis E. Rigid internal fixation for treatment of infected mandibular frac-tures. J Oral Maxillofac Surg 1992; 50:434–443.

[64] Koury M. Complications of mandibular fractures. In: Kaban LB, Pogrell AH, Perrot D, eds. Complications in Oral and Maxillofacial Surgery. Philadelphia: WB. Saun-ders, 1997:121–146.

[65] Passeri LA, Ellis E, Sinn DP. Relationship of substance abuse to complications with mandibular fractures. Journal of Oral and Maxillofacial Surgery 1993;51: 22-25

[66] Moulton-Barrett R, Rubinstein AJ, Salzhauer MA et al. Complications of mandibular fractures. Annals of Plastic Surgery 1998;41 :258-263

[67] Thaller SR. Management of mandibular fractures. Arch Otolaryngol Head Neck Surg 1994; 120:44.

[68] Izuka T, Lindquist C. Sensory disturbances associated with rigid internal fixation of mandibular fractures. J Oral Maxillofac Surg 1991; 49:1264.

[69] Marchena JM, Padwa BL, Kaban LB. Sensory abnormalities associated with mandib-ular fractures: incidence and natural history. J Oral Maxillofac Surg 1998; 56:822–825.

[70] Dingman RO, Grabb WC. Surgical anatomy of the mandibular ramus of the facial nerve based on the dissection of 100 facial halves. Plast Reconstr Surg 1962; 29:266.

[71] Brusati R, Paini P. Facial nerve injury secondary to lateral displacement of the man-dibular ramus. Plast Reconstr Surg 1978; 62(5):728–733.

[72] Al-Kayat A, Bramley PA. A modified pre-auricular approach to the temporomandib-ular joint and malar arch. Br J Oral Maxillofac Surg 1979.

[73] Zuniga JR. Advances in microsurgical nerve repair. Journal of Oral and Maxillofacial Surgery 1993; 51 (suppl I): 62-68

[74] Thurmuller P, Dodson TB, Kaban LB. Nerve injuries associated with facial trauma: natural history, management, and outcomes of repair. Oral and Maxillofacial Surgery Clinics of North America 2001; 13(2): 283-293

Advanced Maxillofacial Distraction Osteogenesis: State-of-the-Art

Chapter 3

Distraction Osteogenesis

Hossein Behnia, Azita Tehranchi and Golnaz Morad

Additional information is available at the end of the chapter

1. Introduction

Distraction osteogenesis (DO) is defined as the formation of new bone between the vascular surfaces of osteotomized bone segments, separated gradually by distraction forces. [1] The incipient concept of distraction osteogenesis, as first described for correction of limb length discrepancies by Codivilla [2] in 1905, represented an osteotomized femur subjected to repeated forces of traction and counter-traction. This technique achieved a length increase of 3 to 8 cm; an amount that surpassed that attainable by other methods common at that time. Codivilla asserted that confronting the resistance of the muscles surrounding a bone is inevitable if the discrepancies are to be corrected. Abbott and Saunders later used the technique for elongation of tibia. [3] Distraction osteogenesis proved advantageous over other conventional methods for management of bone defects, particularly bone grafting, in that it provided simultaneous expansion of the functional soft tissue matrix, referred to as *distraction histogenesis*. [1] The method however, remained undeveloped until it resurged in 1950s by Ilizarov, leading to several successful endeavors increasing the length of the extremities. In 1992, McCarthy [4] expanded the application of distraction osteogenesis to the craniofacial skeleton by attempting to ameliorate mandibular length deficiency in patients with hemifacial microsomia and Nager's syndrome. Accomplishing an average increase of 20 mm in the mandibular length in these preliminary cases, craniofacial DO rendered promising insights for treatment of craniofacial skeletal abnormalities. Hitherto, a plethora of treatment protocols and modalities have evolved in order to improve the outcomes of craniofacial DO.

2. The biology of distraction osteogenesis

Distraction osteogenesis initiates by surgically simulating bone fractures via osteotomy of the deficient bone. Normal fracture healing occurs through a cascade of molecular and cellular events triggered in response to injury. Formation of hematoma followed by chondrogenesis and angiogenesis eventually leads to the formation of hard callus by means of intramembranous and endochondral ossification. The resultant woven bone subsequently remodels into a more mature lamellar bone to restore the strength and function of the organ. [5], [6] During distraction osteogenesis however, the application of mechanical forces to the bone segments alters the repair process of the osteotomized bone segments, characteristic of fracture healing, to a regenerative process. [5] Evaluation of mechanotransduction mechanisms has demonstrated that tensile forces increase the expression of bone morphogenic proteins by osteoblasts and stimulate intramembranous bone formation. [7] This regenerative effect of gradual traction on tissue growth was originally designated by Ilizarov as the Law of Tension-Stress. [8] The process of distraction osteogenesis incorporates 3 major phases. The *Latency* phase is the period Which starts immediately subsequent to the creation of osteotomy and lasts till the commencement of distraction. This delay allows for tissue organization and formation of callus which bridges the gap between the two osteotomized bone surfaces. [5], [9], [10] Aronson et al conducted an animal study to test the outcome of different latency durations on bone regenerations. [11] Contrasting to other concurrent studies, it was observed that bone formation was most reliable when no latency period was considered prior to distraction; hence the suggestion that latency phase may not be essential. A recent study appraising the benefits of the latency period on the outcomes of dentoalveolar DO proved that although a latency period did not enhance the amount and density of the newly formed bone, it slightly increased bone maturation. However, it was assumed that despite the minor effect of the latency period on the regenerated bone, this phase may be crucial for soft tissue regeneration. [12] Regardless of the existing controversy on the importance of the latency phase, a review on the corresponding literature demonstrated that a 5-7 day latency period is the most recommendable protocol for the various indications of craniofacial DO. [1]The second phase known as the *Distraction* period is characterized by the application of distraction forces. Histologically, this phase begins with configuration of a Fibrous Inter-Zone (FIZ) at which dense fibers of collagen demonstrate a longitudinal arrangement parallel to the direction of the distraction forces. In between the collagen bundles osteoblastic activity creates a zone of Micro-Column Formation (MCF). The two ends of the FIZ are characterized by areas of primary mineralization, thus dubbed as Primary Mineralization Front (PMF). [5], [10], [13] The distraction phase continues with active synthesis of fibrous tissue in central areas and active mineralization at the ends, till the acquired amount of elongation is gained. [14] As the major features of the distraction phase, Ilizarov underscored the significance of the rate and rhythm of distraction forces on the quality and quantity of the newly regenerated bone. The rate and the rhythm, respectively defined as the speed and the frequency of the applied distraction forces were assessed in an animal study. The results, reported in 1989, suggested distraction of 1 mm per day applied as 0.25 mm per 6 hours as the ideal distraction rate and rhythm for limb elongation. This was while slower distraction rates led to premature consolidation of the bone and faster distraction was accompanied by hindrance of osteogenesis. Moreover, he claimed that more satisfying results were obtained when distraction forces were applied with higher frequencies. [15] The current standard protocols of craniofacial DO seem to apply distraction forces at a rate of 1 mm per day 2-3 times. Nevertheless, these features may be altered in different patients. [1] Subsequent to the cessation of distraction, the third phase, designated as the *Consolidation* phase begins. This stage of distraction osteogenesis is distinguished by the growth of mineralization in a centripetal pattern. Moreover, transverse bridging connects the micro-columns of bone in the IFZ, leaving a honeycomb appearance. By the end of this phase, bone is being remodeled into a more mature lamellar bone, strong enough to function. [10] The duration of this period can be determined based on the amount of distraction. One month consolidation has been suggested for each centimeter of distraction. [16]

3. Mandibular distraction osteogenesis

The primary attempts for mandibular distraction osteogenesis date back to the 1970s when animal studies were designed to restore surgically shortened canine mandibles via gradual distraction. [17], [18] McCarthy et al were the first to apply gradual distraction for lengthening the human mandible. [4] The preliminary report of their study presented four children who underwent unilateral and bilateral mandibular expansion for management of unilateral microsomia and Nager's syndrome, respectively; 18 to 24 mm of mandibular distraction was achieved. Common indications for mandibular distraction are summarized in Table 1.

Syndromic
Goldenhar Syndrome
Pierre Robin Sequence
Treacher Collins Syndrome
Nager's Syndrome
Non-Syndromic mandibular hypoplasia (Unilateral/ Bilateral)
Retrognathia
Narrow mandible
Hemifacial Microsomia
Obstructive Sleep Apnea
Temporomandibular joint
Lack of TMJ translation
TMJ Ankylosis
Segmental bone defects
Alveolar Deficiencies

Table 1. Common indications for mandibular distraction osteogenesis

3.1. Mandibular lengthening

Mandibular hypoplasia, a condition associated with length deficiency in the mandibular ramus or/ and body, is a manifestation of impairment of mandibular growth caused by syndromic or non-syndromic congenital conditions or as a result of trauma. Depending on the severity of the deficiency, mild to severe esthetic and functional problems arise which obligate intervention. Mandibular hypoplasia has been traditionally managed by bone grafting, orthognathic surgery, and orthodontic therapy. These treatment approaches may contribute to considerable morbidity and unsatisfactory results in many situations, not to mention instances in which treatment appears unfeasible. The advent of craniofacial distraction osteogenesis has provided an alternative treatment modality to eliminate the shortcomings of conventional protocols for management of this craniofacial discrepancy. [4] In correction of mandibular hypoplasia in angle's class II patients where great amounts of advancement (> 10 mm) are required, DO has shown promising results with negligible relapse. This is probably due to the simultaneous expansion of the surrounding soft tissue. [19] In comparison, the bilateral sagittal split osteotomy, the most common treatment choice, not only provides less stable results with advancements larger than 6 mm, but is also likely to be accompanied by serious adverse events, namely neurosensory disturbance of inferior alveolar nerve and disorders of the temporomandibular joint. [20], [21] On the other hand, bone grafting is another common choice of treatment for severe hypoplastic mandibles. [22], [23] Yet, the procedure seems not to be very desirable, since it may be associated with donor site morbidity and resorption of the graft. Another important indication for mandibular distraction osteogenesis is a lack of condylar translation. In growing patients with mandibular hypoplasia in whom condylar translations occurs normally during mandibular movements, functional orthodontic treatment may be of greater merit for restoration of the deficiency. Nevertheless, DO is a technique-sensitive procedure and demands patient compliance. Therefore, until randomized controlled trials have proved it beneficial over other treatment options for mandibular hypoplasia, it remains an alternative rather than a replacement for the existing treatment modalities. [20], [21] A variety of distraction devices have been designed and introduced for clinical implications; each associated with pros and cons. Extraoral distractors which are fixed in place by transcutaneous pins, are generally easier to manipulate and allow for multidirectional distraction. However, the psychosocial problems consequent to the presence of the device as well as facial scarring led to the emergence of intraoral distractors. [24], [25] McCarthy introduced the first intraoral distraction device in 1995. [26] Intraoral distractors are of three types: tooth-borne, bone-borne and hybrid distractors. [25] Finite element analysis of intraoral distraction devices demonstrated the hybrid type to be the most stable under masticatory loads, while tooth-borne distractors were the most reliable in transferring the expansion to the bone. [27] The morbidity associated with bone-borne devices appear to be higher than tooth-borne distractors. [28] While tooth-borne devices seem beneficial as they facilitate subsequent tooth movement, concerns such as greater mandibular expansion at the alveolar section comparing to the basal bone may arise with this type of distractor. [25] Shetye et al demonstrated that application of intraoral distractors may be associated with higher incidence of minor adverse events, with no effect on treatment outcome. This is while the occurrence of major incidents is more likely when extraoral distraction devices are used. [29] Mandibular hypoplasia is generally divided into two groups of unilateral and bilateral hypoplasia. A meta-analysis of mandibular distraction osteogenesis demonstrated the most common indication for unilateral DO to be hemifacial/craniofacial microsomia. [30] Unilateral craniofacial microsomia is a genetic disorder that affects the derivatives of the first and the second brachial arch and is initially characterized by abnormal growth of the mandibular ramus. The asymmetric growth of the mandible may gradually affect the growth of the surrounding structures, a fact that encourages surgeons to begin treating patients at early ages. The resultant facial asymmetry has been corrected via unilateral DO particularly in growing children. [31], [32] The authors analyzed the posteroanterior cephalometric changes subsequent to unilateral distraction osteogenesis in 10 patients. [33] Improvements in the piriform angle, intergonial angle, and the occlusal cant revealed the influence of the treatment on the maxillary and midfacial growth. It is highly suggested that the treatment be continued with functional orthodontic therapy in growing children. Functional appliances can act to obtain symmetry during growth. We have performed the combination of distraction osteogenesis and functional orthodontic therapy in a group of our patients. [34] It is advisable that the patient be followed until the end of growth and if necessary the functional orthodontic therapy be continued.

3.1.1. Lengthening for asymmetry

Case 1

An 8-year-old male patient with a history of right condylar trauma at birth presented with facial asymmetry, cant of the occlusal plane, deviation of the midline, and a deep-bite malocclusion (Figure 1-A, B, C). A horizontal osteotomy was made at the body of the right ramus below the mandibular foramen and a custom-made unidirectional extraoral distractor was fixed in place (Figure 1-D, E). Following a 7-day latency period, the distractor was activated at a rate of 1mm/ day. Distraction was stopped after the ramus was elongated by 22 mm (Figure 1-F). Subsequent to removal of the distractor a hybrid functional appliance was used to manage the posterior right open-bite created as a result of mandibular lengthening (Figure 1-G, H). Functional therapy continued for 3 years when fixed orthodontic therapy was initiated in order to restore the position of impacted left canine (Figure 1-I, J).

3.1.2. Unilateral mandibular hypoplasia

Case 2

A 6-year-old male patient with a history of trauma at age 2, presented with facial asymmetry and midline deviation due to unilateral mandibular hypoplasia (Figure 2-A, B). A horizontal osteotomy was done in the right ramus and a unidirectional intraoral distractor (KLS Martin, Tuttlingen, Germany) was fixed in place (Figure 2-C). Distraction was initiated with an oblique vector (Figure 2-D). Consequently, along with a posterior open bite, the teeth were deviated to the opposite side to a considerable extent (Figure 2-E). This was corrected via cross elastic traction (Figure 2-F). The patient was followed during growth and no deviation or facial asymmetry occurred; hence no need for further orthodontic treatment.

3.1.3. Hemifacial microsomia

Case 3

A 9-year-old male patient with hemifacial microsomia type 2 A was planned to receive distraction osteogenesis for treatment of facial asymmetry (Figure 3-A, B). Mandibular ramus

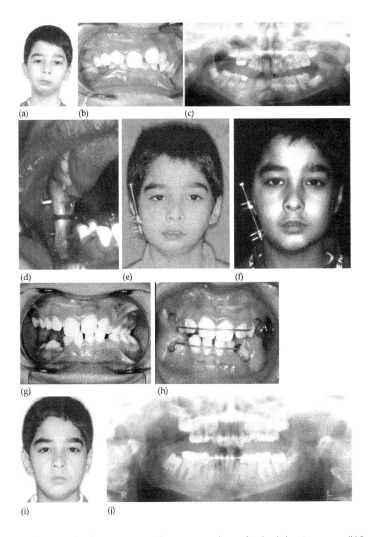

Figure 1. (a) Pre-distraction facial appearance. Facial asymmetry and cant of occlusal plane is apparent. (b) Pre-distraction intraoral view. (c) Panoramic view. (d) Horizontal osteotomy was made at the body of the right ramus below the mandibular foramen. (e) A custom-made unidirectional extraoral distractor was fixed in place. (f) Ramus was elongated by 22 mm. (g) The posterior open-bite was created at the right side as a result of mandibular lengthening. (h) A hybrid functional appliance was used to manage the posterior right open-bite. (i) Facial appearance 3 years post-distraction. (j) Panoramic view 3 years post-distraction.

was elongated using an extraoral distractor. Following a 2-month consolidation period, the distractor was removed. Orthodontic functional therapy was started to correct the posterior open bite (Figure 3-C, D). Orthodontic therapy was continued for 5 years (Figure 3-E, F).

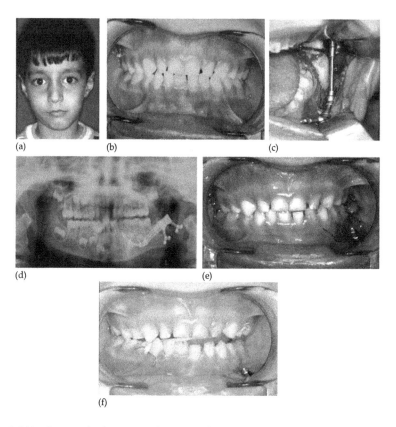

Figure 2. (a) Pre-distraction facial appearance demonstrates facial asymmetry due to childhood trauma. (b) Intraoral view shows midline deviation. (c) A horizontal osteotomy was made at the body of the right ramus and an intraoral distractor was fixed in place. (d) Distraction was initiated with an oblique vector. (e) Post-distraction intraoral view. Teeth were deviated to the opposite side. (f) Deviation was corrected via cross elastic traction.

3.1.4. Hemifacial microsomia

Case 4

A 17 year-old female patient with hemifacial microsomia presented with facial asymmetry and midline deviation to the right. The right maxillary canine was impacted (Figure 4-A-E). Pre-distraction orthodontic therapy included maxillary expansion and repositioning the impacted canine into the arch (Figure 4-F, G). Subsequently, unilateral osteotomy in the ramus was performed and an extraoral distraction device was fixed in place. With a rate of 1mm per day, distraction was continued until adequate elongation was obtained (Figure 4-H-K). Fixed orthodontic treatment was ongoing during the consolidation period (Figure 4-L). Final maxillary and mandibular arch coordination was achieved through bimaxillary orthognathic surgery (Figure 4-M-S).

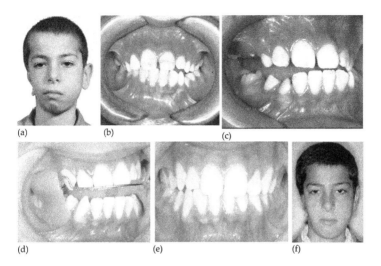

Figure 3. (a) Pre-distraction facial asymmetry due to hemifacial microsomia. (b) Pre-distraction intraoral view. (c) Post-distraction intraoral view. Unilateral posterior open was created. (d) Orthodontic functional therapy was started to correct the posterior open bite. (e) Five years post-distraction intraoral view. (f) Facial appearance 5 years post-distraction.

3.1.5. Facial asymmetry

Case 5

A 13-year-old female patient presented with mandibular deformity due to left condylar ankylosis (Figure 5-A). The patient had received a costochondral graft at age 6 and the function of the joint was restored (Figure 5-B). The remaining facial asymmetry was planned to be resolved via distraction osteogenesis. Using an extraoral custom-made distraction device, the left ramus was elongated by 18 mm (Figure 5-C). The resultant posterior open bite was corrected via 3 years of hybrid functional therapy followed by fixed orthodontic treatment (Figure 5-D, E, F).

3.1.6. Mandibular asymmetry due to condylar ankylosis

Case 6

A 16-year-old female patient presented with mandibular asymmetry due to left condylar ankylosis (Figure 6-A, B). At age 8, the patient had undergone a condylectomy procedure for treatment of the condylar ankylosis. She was then a candidate for distraction osteogenesis. Elongation of the left ramus (20 mm) was achieved by an extraoral distraction device (Leibinger Multiguide, Freiburg, Germany) (Figure 6-C, D). Eight months following removal of the distractor, the patient was orthodontically prepared for an orthognathic surgery. The surgery included Le Fort I and bilateral sagittal split osteotomies as well as genioplasty. A normal class I occlusion was obtained (Figure 6-E, F).

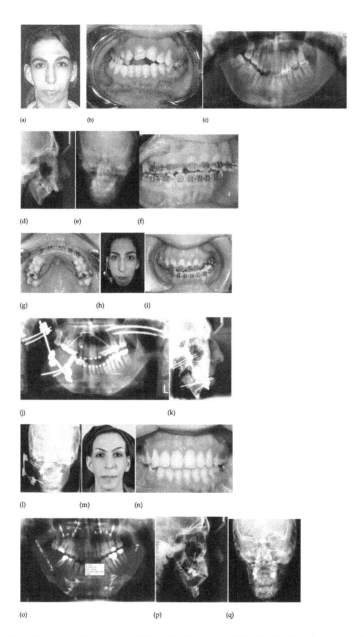

Figure 4. (a) Pre-distraction facial asymmetry. (b) Pre-distraction intraoral view. (c) Pre-distraction panoramic view. (d) Pre-distraction lateral cephalometric view. (e) Pre-distraction posteroanterior (PA) cephalometric view. (f) Orthodon-

tics included maxillary expansion. (g) The impacted canine was brought into the arch. (h) Post-distraction facial appearance. (i) Post-distraction intraoral view. (j) Post-distraction panoramic view. (k) Post-distraction lateral cephalometric view. (l) Post-distraction PA cephalometric view. (m) Post-orthognathic surgery facial appearance. (n) Post-orthognathic surgery intraoral view. (o) Post-orthognathic surgery panoramic radiograph. (p) Lateral cephalometric radiograph. (q) Post-orthognathic surgery PA cephalometric radiograph.

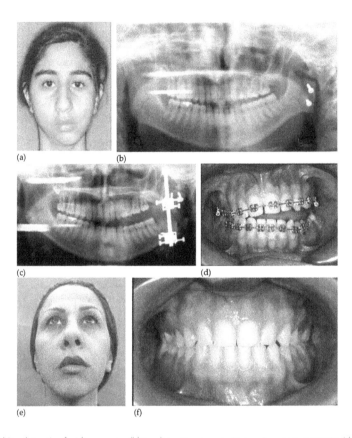

Figure 5. (a) Pre-distraction facial asymmetry. (b) Pre-distraction panoramic view. Bone screws remained from a previous costochondral bone graft can be observed. (c) Immediate post-distraction panoramic view. Mandibular ramus elongated by 18 mm. (d) Posterior open bite was corrected via functional therapy and fixed orthodontic therapy. (e) Six years post-distraction facial appearance. (f) Normal occlusion was obtained.

3.2. Bilateral hypoplasia

Similar to unilateral mandibular hypoplasia, several etiologies are documented for bilateral hypoplasia including syndromic conditions, condylar fracture due to trauma, and class II malocclusion. Along with undesirable facial appearance and disorders in the masticatory system, micrognathia which itself may be symmetric or asymmetric, can cause mild to lethal

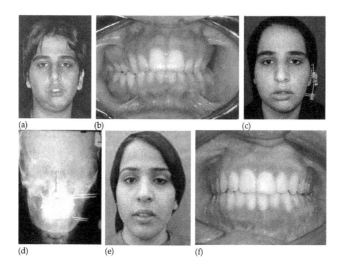

Figure 6. (a) Pre-distraction facial appearance. (b) Pre-distraction intraoral view. (c) Extraoral distractor was used for mandibular lengthening. (d) Left ramus was elongated by 20 mm. (e) Two years post-distraction facial appearance. Orthognathic surgery has been performed. (f) Normal occlusion has been obtained.

degrees of airway obstruction. [35] Havlik and Bartlett [36] as well as Moore and co-workers [37] were the first to apply distraction osteogenesis for management of micrognathia. A meta-analysis indicated Pierre Robin sequence as the most common condition treated with bilateral DO. [30] Pierre Robin syndrome is a congenital anomaly characterized as a triad of micrognathia, glossoptosis, and cleft palate. [38] Obstructive sleep apnea; recognized in severe degrees of the syndrome, implicates intervention at early ages. Severe airway obstruction which may also be a manifestation of temporomandibular joint ankylosis [39] is traditionally treated with tracheotomy. This invasive intervention although remains to be the gold standard, has been associated with considerable morbidity. [40] Mandibular DO allows for early treatment in neonates and infants. It is noteworthy that despite the promising results accomplished with DO at early ages [40]- [42], long-term follow-ups are required to evaluate the stability of the outcomes.

3.2.1. Severe mandibular deficiency

Case 7

A 6-year-old boy presented with severe mandibular deficiency. The patient suffered from obstructive sleep apnea (Figure 7-A-F). Prior to distraction osteogenesis, orthodontic treatment was done and included maxillary arch expansion with a quad-helix appliance followed by application of an anterior bite plate (Figure G). Subsequently, bilateral distraction osteogenesis was performed via extraoral multi-guide distraction devices (Leibinger, Freiburg, Germany). The amount of elongation obtained at the end of the distraction phase was about 32 mm;

though not equal on both sides (Figure H-J). Obstructive sleep apnea was completely resolved in this patient. Treatment was continued with functional orthodontic therapy; however, the patient was only followed for 2 years (Figure K-P).

3.2.2. Mandibular deficiency

Case 8

A 14-year-old patient presented with skeletal class II malocclusion and severe deep bite (Figure 8-A, B). The deficiency was planned to be corrected by distraction osteogenesis. Bilateral horizontal osteotomies were made in the body of the ramus. Unidirectional intraoral distractors (KLS Martin, Tuttlingen, Germany) were fixed in place (Figure 8-C). Following mandibular lengthening for 20 mm, an anterior open bite was created which could be attributable to improper distraction vector, a common adverse event with unidirectional distraction devices (Figure 8-D). This problem was solved by elastic traction (Figure 8-E) and normal occlusion was obtained. The patient has now been followed for 8 years (Figure 8-F, G).

3.3. Mandibular widening

Transverse mandibular deficiency is a common clinical problem, diagnosed by a narrow, V-shaped arch and anterior dental crowding. This problem may occur as an isolated condition, a component of certain syndromes [43], or a consequence of symphyseal fracture and tissue loss. [25], [44] Depending on the amount of the deficiency, various treatment protocols are available for mandibular arch expansion. The use of Arch wires, Schwarz plates, lingual arches and functional appliances has been hampered to some extent by the limited stability of the accomplished results. On the other hand, tooth extraction or interdental stripping, more commonly indicated for adult patients, may not provide adequate space in severe cases. [44], [45] Management of extreme transverse deficiencies was conventionally achieved via osteotomy and placement of bone grafts. Attempting to rectify the possible adverse events of bone grafting, Guerrero first used symphyseal distraction osteogenesis for mandibular widening and called it "rapid surgical mandibular expansion". [46] This technique holds promising potential for expansion of the mandibular basal bone. More predictable results can be obtained in a shorter treatment period. Yet, the probable relapse of the treatment gains is a major concern for surgeons. The possibility of teeth proclination, nonhomogeneous dental and skeletal expansion, as well as device-related difficulties should also be taken into consideration. [47] Based on the literature, symphyseal distraction osteogenesis has been suggested for patients above 12 years old. [1] Chung and Tae evaluated dental stability in an average 1.5 year follow-up duration subsequent to symphyseal distraction osteogenesis. By following the changes of 13 landmarks on study models, it was demonstrated that the total amount of surgical expansion did not decrease by relapse. [47] Both extraoral and intraoral distraction devices can be used for symphyseal distraction osteogenesis. Intraoral devices are more esthetically appealing. Though, as suggested by Kita et al, when extremely narrow mandibles are to be expanded, placement of intraoral devices may not be feasible due to inadequate space. Moreover, the design of intraoral distractors does not allow for large amounts of expansion. Kita et al used symphyseal distraction osteogenesis via extraoral devices to treat extreme transverse man-

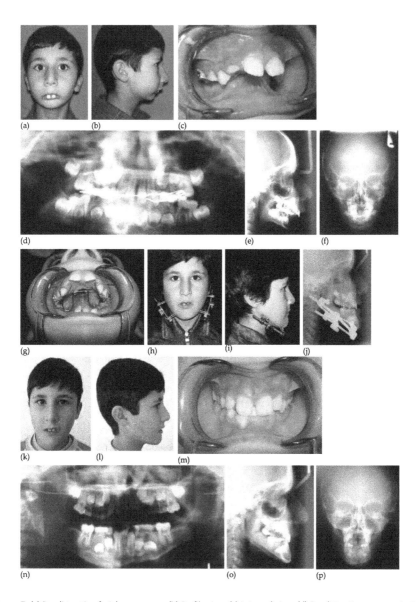

Figure 7. (a) Pre-distraction facial appearance. (b) Profile view. (c) Intraoral view. (d) Pre-distraction panoramic view. (e) Pre-distraction lateral cephalometric view. (f) Pre-distraction posteroanterior cephalometric view. (g) Pre-distraction orthodontic treatment included maxillary expansion via a quad-helix appliance. (h) Post-distraction facial appearance. (i) Profile view. (j) Lateral cephalometric view. (k) Two years post-distraction appearance. (l) Profile. (m) Intraoral view. (n) Two years post-distraction panoramic view. (o) Post-distraction lateral cephalogram. (p) Two years post-distraction PA cephalogram.

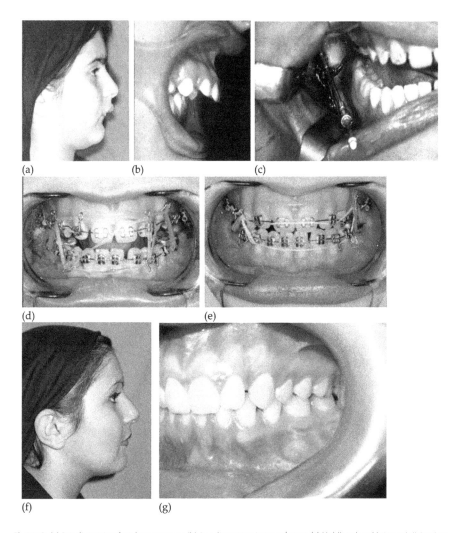

Figure 8. (a) Pre-distraction facial appearance. (b) Pre-distraction intraoral view. (c) Unidirectional intraoral distractors were fixed in place. (d) Following mandibular lengthening for 20 mm, an anterior open bite was created. (e) Anterior open bite was corrected by elastic traction. (f) Eight years post-distraction facial appearance. (g) Intraoral view.

dibular deficiencies in patients with hypoglossia-hypodactyly syndrome. [43]A plethora of investigations and modifications have attributed to enhanced efficiency of mandibular distraction osteogenesis. Yet, the technique is not exempt of adverse events. Diverse rates of incidence have been reported for different mandibular distraction osteogenesis procedures. Shetye et al [29] classified the potential adverse events associated with mandibular DO into three groups: minor incidents indicated those with no influence on the outcome. Moderate and major incidents were both defined as events that result in undesirable outcome and can or cannot be resolved via invasive procedures, respectively. Their 16 year follow-up of 141 patients who underwent mandibular DO for unilateral or bilateral mandibular lengthening demonstrated that minor and moderate incidents were reported in 26.99% and 20.35%, respectively; while in only 5.31% of patients did major events occur. The majority of major incidents included TMJ ankylosis and derangements as well as fibrous union. Nevertheless, taken all the above-mentioned complications into considerations, investigators seem to be unanimous in the safety of distraction osteogenesis.

3.4. Maxillary distraction osteogenesis

The Principles of distraction osteogenesis have been applied for correction of transverse and sagittal discrepancies of the maxilla and the midface associated with orofacial clefts and several syndromes. Midfacial distraction osteogenesis was first evaluated in animal studies performed on sheep [48] and dogs [49]. A preliminary human report of maxillary and midfacial advancement through the application of a distraction device was published by Cohen et al in 1997. [50] Two children with cleft lip and palate, midfacial hypoplasia, and class III malocclusion underwent treatment with distraction osteogenesis. Up to 11 mm advancement of the midfacial complex was achieved in both patients. Two years later, Mommaerts introduced a technique for maxillary expansion using a transpalatal distractor. [51] In comparison to rapid palatal expansion, the treatment protocol most frequently used for maxillary expansion, palatal distraction osteogenesis was asserted to eliminate particular adverse events such as alveolar bending, tooth tipping, buccal cortex fenestration, and relapse. Common indications for maxillary and midface distraction osteogenesis are summarized in Table 2.

Orofacial Clefts
Craniosynostosis
Crouzon's Syndrome
Apert's Syndrome
Pfeiffer Syndrome
Midface deficiencies of other causes
Alveolar deficiencies

Table 2. Common indications for maxillary and midface distraction osteogenesis.

3.5. Maxillary and midfacial advancement

The majority of cleft lip and palate patients suffer from degrees of maxillary hypoplasia, either as a primary manifestation of the cleft or secondary to attempts for cleft repair. This often complex discrepancy is conventionally corrected through a series of surgeries including different osteotomies. The inception of distraction osteogenesis for advancement of maxillary-midface in cleft patients brought new insight into the treatment of these patients. A meta-analysis of conventional osteotomies and distraction osteogenesis, along with many similarities between the two techniques, suggested distraction osteogenesis to be advantageous for it eliminates the need for bone grafts. [52] Moreover, it was demonstrated that most protocols postponed treatment with conventional osteotomies until growth was completed. In contrast, distraction osteogenesis was more frequently performed in growing patients; although, overcorrection was recommended to preclude relapse. Different types of extraoral and intraoral distractors have been established for maxillary distraction osteogenesis. Extraoral distractors have the capacity for multidirectional maxillary advancement and the vectors can be changed during the process. [53] Yet, many patients have difficulty accepting extraoral devices primarily due to the unappealing appearance and discomfort. [54] Moreover, the external position of these devices makes them prone to loosening and fracture following an accidental trauma. [53] Rigid external distraction (RED) device is fixed to the cranium. This allows for protection of maxillary teeth comparing to other types of extraoral devices which are anchored to the maxilla. [54] The stability of maxillary advancement with RED was evaluated in a 3-year prospective study. To avoid the possible interference of growth in the outcomes, the study was performed on adult patients. The relapse was reported to be 22% after 3 years. [55] Internal distractors cause less psychosocial problems for the patient and are less likely to be loosened or displaced during the distraction period or following traumatic forces. Moreover, being more easily tolerated by patients, an internal device can be maintained during the consolidation phase for as long as deemed necessary for prevention of relapse. [53], [54], [56] Nevertheless, installation of intraoral distractors may not be always feasible due to inadequate space. In addition, intraoral distractors provide unidirectional bone movement; hence demanding precise positioning. [53] Complications such as fracture and collapse of the cleft alveolar bone has been reported with intraoral devices used for Le Fort I distraction. [56] Picard et al described a rigid internal device (RID) with the ability to provide unrestricted lengthening for total or segmental advancement of the maxilla. In 19 syndromic, cleft, and traumatic patients treated with this distractor, an average advancement of 9.6 mm was achieved. [54] A retrospective study comparing extraoral and intraoral distractors for midface advancement in syndromic patients demonstrated no significant difference regarding the complication rate and amount of lengthening between the two types. Accordingly, both distractors were asserted to be safe and it was suggested that choosing a device be individualized based on each patients needs and toleration. [53]Mild to moderate cases of maxillary hypoplasia which were traditionally corrected via Le Fort I osteotomy, have been successfully treated with anterior maxillary distraction osteogenesis. [57] Le Fort I osteotomy shows a negative impact on velopharyngeal competence and speech while this problem is rarely seen with anterior maxillary distraction osteogenesis. [57] Nonetheless, more severe cases may necessitate Le Fort I distraction.

3.5.1. Cleft lip and palate and class III malocclusion

Case 9

A 17-year-old female patient with cleft lip and palate presented with a class III malocclusion and anterior and posterior cross bite (Figure 9 A-C). Following pre-distraction orthodontic treatment, maxillary advancement was performed through Le Fort I osteotomy and RED device (KLS Martin, Figure 9-D). Maxilla was advanced by 18 mm (Figure 9-E, F). Orthodontic treatment continued for a year. Meanwhile, the patient received a removable partial prosthesis to replace the anterior missing teeth. Subsequently, the patient underwent rhinoplasty and primary lip repair (Figure 9-G-J). The procedures for lip repair are still ongoing.

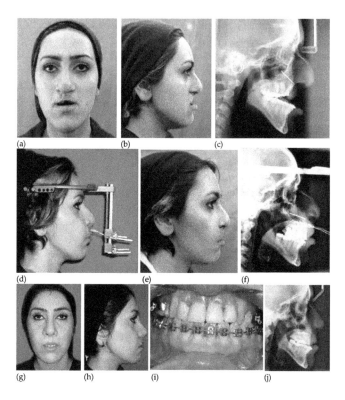

Figure 9. (a) Pre-distraction appearance. (b) Profile view. (c) Lateral cephalometric view. (d) Maxillary distraction osteogenesis was performed using an RED device. (e) Post-distraction facial appearance. (f) Post-distraction lateral cephalometric view. (g) Two years post-distraction facial appearance. (h) Profile. (i) Intraoral view. (j) Lateral cephalometric view.

Distraction osteogenesis has also proved valuable for treatment of patients affected with craniosynostosis. This condition caused as a result of premature fusion of cranial sutures is a clinical feature of particular syndromes such as Crouzon, Apert, and Pfeiffer. In the severe expression of these syndromes, it may be crucial to initiate treatment as early as 1 year of age. [58] Le Fort III and monobloc osteotomies are frequently used for management of craniosynostosis. [59] During the recent years, distraction osteogenesis has become popular for correction of syndromic maxillary hypoplasia. The amount of advancement of midface that can be achieved by distraction osteogenesis is generally greater than the amount obtained by conventional osteotomies such as Le Fort III and monobloc osteotomy. [60] Long-term follow ups of syndromic patients who underwent maxillary-midface advancement with distraction osteogenesis have proved the stability of the results. [59], [61], [62]

3.6. Maxillary expansion

Maxillary transverse deficiency is a condition associated with anterior and posterior dental crowding, unilateral or bilateral cross-bite, as well as TMJ and respiratory problems. Expansion of maxillary bone during growth is usually feasible through orthodontic treatments. However, with skeletal maturation, a combination of surgical and orthodontic techniques may be inevitable in order to accomplish adequate expansion. When the condition is accompanied with cleft lip and palate, it poses even greater challenges for treatment. Treatment of maxillary constriction can be performed by means of Le Fort I osteotomy and expansion. This protocol allows for multidirectional expansion of the maxillary complex; however, the resistance of the palatal fibromucosa diminishes the stability of the results. Another treatment option established for this deformity is surgically assisted rapid maxillary expansion (SARME). This technique eliminates soft tissue resistance via distraction histogenesis and can be based upon either tooth-borne or bone-borne devices. Tooth-borne distractors transfer forces to the teeth, leading to tooth-related adverse events such as root resorption, tooth tipping, and cortical fenestration. In contrast, bone-borne devices; first introduced by Mommaerts as a transpalatal distractor (TPD), are exempt of these undesirable effects for they directly apply forces to the bone. [63], [64] Application of bone-borne distractors becomes of paramount importance particularly when insufficient tooth support exists due to tooth missing and impaction. [65] Yet, they require a secondary surgery for removal. [63], [64] It is noteworthy that despite the disadvantages commonly considered for tooth-borne device, no considerable difference in dental tipping and stability has been found between tooth-borne and bone-borne maxillary distractors. [64], [66]

3.6.1. Skeletal class III malocclusion and narrow maxilla

Case 10

A 25-year-old female patient presented with dental and skeletal class III malocclusion and a narrow maxilla. Both maxillary and mandibular midlines had a shift to the right side. A 2-mm reverse overjet and anterior and posterior cross bites were present (Figure 10-A-D). Restriction in mandibular movement was found on examination. Treatment plan included SARPE via Smile distractor (Titamed). Transverse distraction was started at a rate of 1mm/ day and continued until 10 mm expansion was achieved (Figure 10-E, F). Post-distraction fixed orthodontic treatment closed the resultant gap between the two central incisors and repositioned the right lateral incisor into the dental arch (Figure 10-G-J).

3.6.2. Maxillary transverse deficiency

Case 11

A 20-year-old male patient presented with a class III malocclusion, maxillary transverse deficiency, severe anterior crowding, anterior open-bite, and bilateral cross-bite (Figure 11-A-

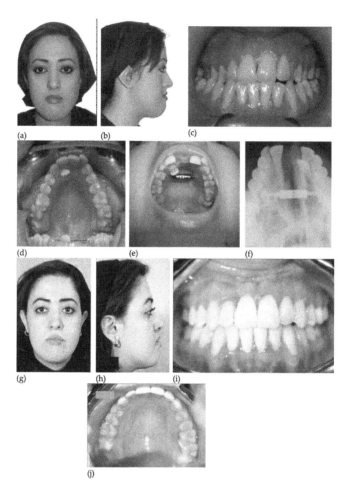

Figure 10. (a) Pre-distraction facial appearance. (b) Profile. (c) Intraoral view. (d) Pre-distraction intraoral view, the right lateral incisor is in a palatal position. (e) Post-distraction intraoral view. Maxilla expanded by 10mm. (f) Post-distraction radiograph. (g) Post-orthodontic treatment facial appearance. (h) Profile. (i) Intraoral view. (j) Post-orthodontic intraoral view. The right lateral incisor is repositioned into the arch.

E). The treatment plan included SARME with a bone-borne distractor followed by orthognathic surgery in order to respectively correct the transverse deficiency and the open bite. An osteotomy was made in the palatal midline, between the roots of the two central incisors and the distraction device (Smile distractor, Titamed) was placed (Figure 11-F-H). Following a 7-day latency period, the distractor was activated at a rate of 1mm/ day. When expansion of 10 mm was achieved, activation was stopped and the device was maintained for a 2-month consolidation period (Figure 11-I). The device was kept for another 4 months until the space created between the central incisors was closed by orthodontic forces. Subsequently, the patient was orthodontically prepared for orthognathic surgery, Le Fort I osteotomy (Figure 11-K). Arch coordination was obtained. The patient is still under orthodontic treatment (Figure 11-L-P). It is worth mentioning that in this patient, alignment of maxillary teeth could have been achieved by extraction of premolars and fixed orthodontic therapy. However, this treatment protocol would impede maxillary and mandibular arch coordination. On the other hand, it is important that the amount of maxillary expansion is proportional to the mandibular arch.

3.7. Alveolar distraction osteogenesis

Alveolar distraction osteogenesis is pre-implant/ pre-prosthetic procedure which tends to restore the alveolar deficiencies and prepare the alveolar ridge for further rehabilitative treatments. Alveolar distraction osteogenesis was first evaluated in an animal model by Block et al. [67] Chin and Toth extended its application to human. [68] Alveolar ridge augmentation is frequently conducted via the use of different types of bone grafts. However, distraction osteogenesis not only decreases the complications and the duration of treatment, but also allows for reconstruction of large defects by simultaneously expanding the surrounding soft tissue. [69] Studies have suggested the amount of newly formed bone resorption prior to implant placement to be greater with onlay bone grafting in comparison to distraction osteogenesis. Peri-implant bone loss was comparable between the two techniques. [70], [71] On the other hand, the amount of augmentation gained with distraction osteogenesis was reported to be significantly greater than that obtained with inlay bone grafts. [72] Depending on the type and the extension of an alveolar defect, distraction osteogenesis may be considered either as an absolute treatment for reconstruction or as an adjunctive therapy along with other bone grafting procedures. Jensen and Block presented a classification of alveolar defects aiming to facilitated treatment planning with alveolar distraction osteogenesis. Accordingly, the more complex a defect, the greater the possibility of requiring bone grafts prior or subsequent to distraction osteogenesis. [73] This treatment modality can also be considered when previous attempts for bone grafting have failed. [74]

3.7.1. Vertical alveolar distraction osteogenesis

The technique of alveolar distraction osteogenesis have been successfully used for enhancing alveolar ridge height. [69], [74]- [81] The majority of studies evaluated the efficiency of distraction osteogenesis in the anterior parts of maxilla and mandible and the amount of obtained augmentation was reported between 5 to 15 mm. Benefits of this method for augmentation of severely atrophic ridges remains to be a matter of controversy. Basal bone fracture and neurosensory complications have been suggested as the two most common problems associated with vertical distraction of atrophic mandibular ridges. [82] Indication of vertical alveolar distraction osteogenesis is therefore limited to areas where 5-7 mm of alveolar bone exists. [83]

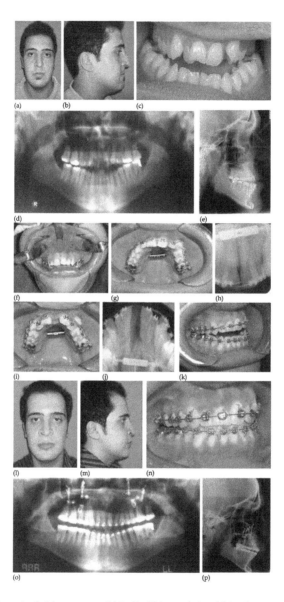

Figure 11. (a) Pre-distraction facial appearance. (b) Profile. (c) Intraoral view. (d) Pre-distraction panoramic view. (e) Pre-distraction lateral cephalometric view. (f) Osteotomy was made in the palatal midline. (g) Palatal distractor in place before activation. (h) Periapical radiography. (i) Two months post-distraction intraoral view. (j) Two months post-distraction occlusal radiograph. (k) Anterior open bite was planned to be corrected via orthognathic surgery. (l) Post-orthognathic surgery facial appearance. (m) Profile. (n) Intraoral view. (o) Post-orthognathic surgery panoramic view. (p) Post-orthognathic cephalometric view.

Distraction devices for alveolar distraction osteogenesis include both extraoral and intraoral devices as well as distraction implants. Extraoral distractors which are mainly positioned subperiosteally in the buccal vestibule, can only be used when a bone height of 6-7 mm is present. Comparing intraoral and extraoral distractors for alveolar distraction osteogenesis, Uckan et al demonstrated that the majority of complications associated with intraoral distractors were related to displacement and fracture of the transport segment. However, interference of the device with the opposing dental arch was considered the most frequent complication with extraoral distractors. [71] Distraction implants initially pose distraction forces to augment the alveolar ridge and are subsequently kept in place to act as a dental implant. These devices have the advantage of eliminating the need for a second surgery for distractor removal. Yet, it is highly likely that the ideal position of the distractor does not correspond to the desirable position of the implant. [81], [83]

3.7.2. Alveolar deficiency

Case 11

A 20 year-old female patient presented with a large bone defect in the anterior mandible due to resection of a central giant cell granuloma (Figure 12-A, B). The patient underwent alveolar distraction osteogenesis. Horizontal osteotomy was performed and an intraoral distractor (KLS Martin) was placed (Figure 12-C, D). Following a 7-day latency phase distraction was initiated at a rate of 1 mm per day. 18mm augmentation was achieved (Figure 12-E). After the consolidation period, the distractor was removed and dental implants were inserted into the regenerated bone. Due to insufficient ridge width, a guided bone regeneration procedure was done to induce bone regeneration over the exposed surfaces of the implants (Figure 12-F). 3 months later, at the second stage of implant surgery inadequate keratinized tissue was compensated by a connective tissue graft from the palate (Figure 12-G-I). Fixed implant-supported prosthesis restored the missing teeth (Figure 12-J).

3.8. Horizontal alveolar distraction osteogenesis

Horizontal alveolar ridge augmentation through distraction osteogenesis demands for extreme preciseness in technique and the design of distractors. The amount of alveolar ridge width increase reported with distraction osteogenesis is 2.5 mm to 7 mm. [84]- [89] Horizontal alveolar distraction can be conducted via simple bone screws to meticulously designed distractors. All devices have a distraction rod in common which is fixed in the cortical lingual/ palatal bone plate and allows for the buccal/ labial movement of the transfer segment. [84] Nevertheless, the intricacy of device positioning as well as the difficulty of performing an osteotomy in a narrow alveolar ridge have greatly restricted the indication of horizontal alveolar distraction osteogenesis. [85] Therefore, in many cases with horizontal alveolar deficiency, bone grafting techniques become advantageous over distraction osteogenesis.

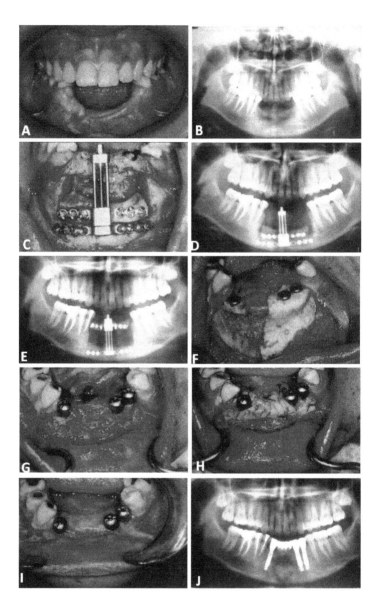

Figure 12. A. Large bone defect in the anterior mandible due to resection of a central giant cell granuloma. Intraoral view. B. Large anterior mandibular defect. Panoramic view. C. Intraoral distractor was placed. D. Panoramic view. E. Post-distraction panoramic view 18mm augmentation was achieved. F. As a result of insufficient ridge width, a guided bone regeneration was done with implant placement. G. Second stage implant surgery, 3 months later. H. Inadequate keratinized tissue was compensated by a connective tissue graft harvested from the palate. I. Two months following the second stage implant surgery. J. Fixed implant-supported prosthesis was placed. Panoramic view.

Acknowledgements

The authors wish to express their sincere gratitude to Dr. Ladan Eslamian; Professor of Department of Orthodontics, School of Dentistry, Shahid Beheshti university of Medical Sciences who took the responsiblity for orthodontic management of one of our patients, presented as case 9.

Author details

Hossein Behnia[1*], Azita Tehranchi[2] and Golnaz Morad[3]

1 Department of Oral and Maxillofacial Surgery, School of Dentistry, Shahid Beheshti University of Medical Sciences, Tehran, Iran

2 Department of Orthodontics, School of Dentistry, Shahid Beheshti University of Medical Sciences, Tehran, Iran

3 Dental Research Center, Shahid Beheshti University of Medical Sciences, Tehran, Iran

References

[1] Swennen G, Schliephake H, Dempf R, Schierle H, Malevez C. Craniofacial distraction osteogenesis: a review of the literature: Part 1: clinical studies. Int J Oral Maxillofac Surg 2001;30(2):89-103.

[2] Codivilla A. The classic: On the means of lengthening, in the lower limbs, the muscles and tissues which are shortened through deformity. 1905. Clin Orthop Relat Res 2008;466(12):2903-9.

[3] Abbott LC, Saunders JB. The Operative Lengthening of the Tibia and Fibula: a Preliminary Report on the Further Development of the Principles and Technic. Ann Surg 1939;110(6):961-91.

[4] McCarthy JG, Schreiber J, Karp N, Thorne CH, Grayson BH. Lengthening the human mandible by gradual distraction. Plast Reconstr Surg 1992;89(1):1-8; discussion 9-10.

[5] Ai-Aql ZS, Alagl AS, Graves DT, Gerstenfeld LC, Einhorn TA. Molecular mechanisms controlling bone formation during fracture healing and distraction osteogenesis. J Dent Res 2008;87(2):107-18.

[6] Marsh DR, Li G. The biology of fracture healing: optimising outcome. Br Med Bull 1999;55(4):856-69.

[7]   Morgan EF, Gleason RE, Hayward LN, Leong PL, Palomares KT. Mechanotransduc-
      tion and fracture repair. J Bone Joint Surg Am 2008;90 Suppl 1:25-30.

[8]   Ilizarov GA. The tension-stress effect on the genesis and growth of tissues. Part I. The
      influence of stability of fixation and soft-tissue preservation. Clin Orthop Relat Res
      1989(238):249-81.

[9]   Fischgrund J, Paley D, Suter C. Variables affecting time to bone healing during limb
      lengthening. Clin Orthop Relat Res 1994(301):31-7.

[10] Aronson J. Experimental and clinical experience with distraction osteogenesis. Cleft
      Palate Craniofac J 1994;31(6):473-81; discussion 81-2.

[11] Aronson J, Shen X. Experimental healing of distraction osteogenesis comparing meta-
      physeal with diaphyseal sites. Clin Orthop Relat Res 1994(301):25-30.

[12] Moore C, Campbell PM, Dechow PC, Ellis ML, Buschang PH. Effects of latency on
      the quality and quantity of bone produced by dentoalveolar distraction osteogenesis.
      Am J Orthod Dentofacial Orthop;140(4):470-8.

[13] Aronson J, Good B, Stewart C, Harrison B, Harp J. Preliminary studies of mineraliza-
      tion during distraction osteogenesis. Clin Orthop Relat Res 1990(250):43-9.

[14] Vauhkonen M, Peltonen J, Karaharju E, Aalto K, Alitalo I. Collagen synthesis and
      mineralization in the early phase of distraction bone healing. Bone Miner 1990;10(3):
      171-81.

[15] Ilizarov GA. The tension-stress effect on the genesis and growth of tissues: Part II.
      The influence of the rate and frequency of distraction. Clin Orthop Relat Res
      1989(239):263-85.

[16] Merloz P. Bone regeneration and limb lengthening. Osteoporos Int;22(6):2033-6.

[17] Michieli S, Miotti B. Lengthening of mandibular body by gradual surgical-orthodon-
      tic distraction. J Oral Surg 1977;35(3):187-92.

[18] Snyder CC, Levine GA, Swanson HM, Browne EZ, Jr. Mandibular lengthening by
      gradual distraction. Preliminary report. Plast Reconstr Surg 1973;51(5):506-8.

[19] Altug-Atac AT, Grayson BH, McCarthy JG. Comparison of skeletal and soft-tissue
      changes following unilateral mandibular distraction osteogenesis. Plast Reconstr
      Surg 2008;121(5):1751-9.

[20] Ow A, Cheung LK. Skeletal stability and complications of bilateral sagittal split os-
      teotomies and mandibular distraction osteogenesis: an evidence-based review. J Oral
      Maxillofac Surg 2009;67(11):2344-53.

[21] Schreuder WH, Jansma J, Bierman MW, Vissink A. Distraction osteogenesis versus
      bilateral sagittal split osteotomy for advancement of the retrognathic mandible: a re-
      view of the literature. Int J Oral Maxillofac Surg 2007;36(2):103-10.

[22] Kaban LB, Moses MH, Mulliken JB. Surgical correction of hemifacial microsomia in the growing child. Plast Reconstr Surg 1988;82(1):9-19.

[23] Padwa BL, Mulliken JB, Maghen A, Kaban LB. Midfacial growth after costochondral graft construction of the mandibular ramus in hemifacial microsomia. J Oral Maxillofac Surg 1998;56(2):122-7; discussion 27-8.

[24] Pereira MA, Luiz de Freitas PH, da Rosa TF, Xavier CB. Understanding distraction osteogenesis on the maxillofacial complex: a literature review. J Oral Maxillofac Surg 2007;65(12):2518-23.

[25] Tae KC, Kang KH, Kim SC. Unilateral mandibular widening with distraction osteogenesis. Angle Orthod 2005;75(6):1053-60.

[26] McCarthy JG, Staffenberg DA, Wood RJ, Cutting CB, Grayson BH, Thorne CH. Introduction of an intraoral bone-lengthening device. Plast Reconstr Surg 1995;96(4): 978-81.

[27] Boccaccio A, Cozzani M, Pappalettere C. Analysis of the performance of different orthodontic devices for mandibular symphyseal distraction osteogenesis. Eur J Orthod; 33(2):113-20.

[28] Raoul G, Wojcik T, Ferri J. Outcome of mandibular symphyseal distraction osteogenesis with bone-borne devices. J Craniofac Surg 2009;20(2):488-93.

[29] Shetye PR, Warren SM, Brown D, Garfinkle JS, Grayson BH, McCarthy JG. Documentation of the incidents associated with mandibular distraction: introduction of a new stratification system. Plast Reconstr Surg 2009;123(2):627-34.

[30] Ow AT, Cheung LK. Meta-analysis of mandibular distraction osteogenesis: clinical applications and functional outcomes. Plast Reconstr Surg 2008;121(3):54e-69e.

[31] Kofod T, Norholt SE, Pedersen TK, Jensen J. Unilateral mandibular ramus elongation by intraoral distraction osteogenesis. J Craniofac Surg 2005;16(2):247-54.

[32] Shetye PR, Grayson BH, Mackool RJ, McCarthy JG. Long-term stability and growth following unilateral mandibular distraction in growing children with craniofacial microsomia. Plast Reconstr Surg 2006;118(4):985-95.

[33] Tehranchi A, Behnia H. Facial symmetry after distraction osteogenesis and orthodontic therapy. Am J Orthod Dentofacial Orthop 2001;120(2):149-53.

[34] Tehranchi A, Behnia H. Treatment of mandibular asymmetry by distraction osteogenesis and orthodontics: a report of four cases. Angle Orthod 2000;70(2):165-74.

[35] Wang X, Wang XX, Liang C, Yi B, Lin Y, Li ZL. Distraction osteogenesis in correction of micrognathia accompanying obstructive sleep apnea syndrome. Plast Reconstr Surg 2003;112(6):1549-57; discussion 58-9.

[36] Havlik RJ, Bartlett SP. Mandibular distraction lengthening in the severely hypoplastic mandible: a problematic case with tongue aplasia. J Craniofac Surg 1994;5(5): 305-10; discussion 11-2.

[37] Moore MH, Guzman-Stein G, Proudman TW, Abbott AH, Netherway DJ, David DJ. Mandibular lengthening by distraction for airway obstruction in Treacher-Collins syndrome. J Craniofac Surg 1994;5(1):22-5.

[38] P R.

[39] Feiyun P, Wei L, Jun C, Xin X, Zhuojin S, Fengguo Y. Simultaneous correction of bilateral temporomandibular joint ankylosis with mandibular micrognathia using internal distraction osteogenesis and 3-dimensional craniomaxillofacial models. J Oral Maxillofac Surg;68(3):571-7.

[40] Senders CW, Kolstad CK, Tollefson TT, Sykes JM. Mandibular distraction osteogenesis used to treat upper airway obstruction. Arch Facial Plast Surg;12(1):11-5.

[41] Scott AR, Tibesar RJ, Lander TA, Sampson DE, Sidman JD. Mandibular distraction osteogenesis in infants younger than 3 months. Arch Facial Plast Surg;13(3):173-9.

[42] Shen W, Jie C, Chen J, Zou J, Ji Y. Mandibular distraction osteogenesis to relieve Pierre Robin severe airway obstruction in neonates: indication and operation. J Craniofac Surg 2009;20 Suppl 2:1812-6.

[43] Kita H, Kochi S, Yamada A, Imai Y, Konno N, Saitou C, et al. Mandibular widening by distraction osteogenesis in the treatment of a constricted mandible and telescopic bite. Cleft Palate Craniofac J 2004;41(6):664-73.

[44] Conley R, Legan H. Mandibular symphyseal distraction osteogenesis: diagnosis and treatment planning considerations. Angle Orthod 2003;73(1):3-11.

[45] Sukurica Y, Gurel HG, Mutlu N. Six year follow-up of a patient treated with mandibular symphyseal distraction osteogenesis. J Craniomaxillofac Surg;38(1):26-31.

[46] Gurrereo.

[47] Chung YW, Tae KC. Dental stability and radiographic healing patterns after mandibular symphysis widening with distraction osteogenesis. Eur J Orthod 2007;29(3): 256-62.

[48] Rachmiel A, Jackson IT, Potparic Z, Laufer D. Midface advancement in sheep by gradual distraction: a 1-year follow-up study. J Oral Maxillofac Surg 1995;53(5):525-9.

[49] Staffenberg DA, Wood RJ, McCarthy JG, Grayson BH, Glasberg SB. Midface distraction advancement in the canine without osteotomies. Ann Plast Surg 1995;34(5): 512-7.

[50] Cohen SR, Burstein FD, Stewart MB, Rathburn MA. Maxillary-midface distraction in children with cleft lip and palate: a preliminary report. Plast Reconstr Surg 1997;99(5):1421-8.

[51] Mommaerts MY. Transpalatal distraction as a method of maxillary expansion. Br J Oral Maxillofac Surg 1999;37(4):268-72.

[52] Cheung LK, Chua HD. A meta-analysis of cleft maxillary osteotomy and distraction osteogenesis. Int J Oral Maxillofac Surg 2006;35(1):14-24.

[53] Meling TR, Hogevold HE, Due-Tonnessen BJ, Skjelbred P. Midface distraction osteogenesis: internal vs. external devices. Int J Oral Maxillofac Surg;40(2):139-45.

[54] Picard A, Diner PA, Galliani E, Tomat C, Vazquez MP, Carls FP. Five years experience with a new intraoral maxillary distraction device (RID). Br J Oral Maxillofac Surg;49(7):546-51.

[55] Aksu M, Saglam-Aydinatay B, Akcan CA, El H, Taner T, Kocadereli I, et al. Skeletal and dental stability after maxillary distraction with a rigid external device in adult cleft lip and palate patients. J Oral Maxillofac Surg;68(2):254-9.

[56] Mitsukawa N, Satoh K, Morishita T. Le Fort I distraction using internal devices for maxillary hypoplasia in patients with cleft lip, palate, and alveolus: complications and their prevention and management. J Craniofac Surg;21(5):1428-30.

[57] Richardson S, Agni NA, Selvaraj D. Anterior maxillary distraction using a tooth-borne device for hypoplastic cleft maxillas-a pilot study. J Oral Maxillofac Surg; 69(12):e542-8.

[58] Marchac A, Arnaud E. Cranium and midface distraction osteogenesis: current practices, controversies, and future applications. J Craniofac Surg;23(1):235-8.

[59] Kuroda S, Watanabe K, Ishimoto K, Nakanishi H, Moriyama K, Tanaka E. Long-term stability of LeFort III distraction osteogenesis with a rigid external distraction device in a patient with Crouzon syndrome. Am J Orthod Dentofacial Orthop;140(4):550-61.

[60] Ko EW, Chen PK, Tai IC, Huang CS. Fronto-facial monobloc distraction in syndromic craniosynostosis. Three-dimensional evaluation of treatment outcome and facial growth. Int J Oral Maxillofac Surg;41(1).20-7.

[61] Fearon JA. Halo distraction of the Le Fort III in syndromic craniosynostosis: a long-term assessment. Plast Reconstr Surg 2005;115(6):1524-36.

[62] Meazzini MC, Allevia F, Mazzoleni F, Ferrari L, Pagnoni M, Iannetti G, et al. Long-term follow-up of syndromic craniosynostosis after Le Fort III halo distraction: a cephalometric and CT evaluation. J Plast Reconstr Aesthet Surg;65(4):464-72.

[63] Cortese A, Savastano M, Savastano G, Claudio PP. One-step transversal palatal distraction and maxillary repositioning: technical considerations, advantages, and long-term stability. J Craniofac Surg;22(5):1714-9.

[64] Seeberger R, Kater W, Schulte-Geers M, Davids R, Freier K, Thiele O. Changes after surgically-assisted maxillary expansion (SARME) to the dentoalveolar, palatal and nasal structures by using tooth-borne distraction devices. Br J Oral Maxillofac Surg; 49(5):381-5.

[65] Verlinden CR, Gooris PG, Becking AG. Complications in transpalatal distraction osteogenesis: a retrospective clinical study. J Oral Maxillofac Surg;69(3):899-905.

[66] Verstraaten J, Kuijpers-Jagtman AM, Mommaerts MY, Berge SJ, Nada RM, Schols JG. A systematic review of the effects of bone-borne surgical assisted rapid maxillary expansion. J Craniomaxillofac Surg;38(3):166-74.

[67] Block MS, Chang A, Crawford C. Mandibular alveolar ridge augmentation in the dog using distraction osteogenesis. J Oral Maxillofac Surg 1996;54(3):309-14.

[68] Chin M, Toth BA. Distraction osteogenesis in maxillofacial surgery using internal devices: review of five cases. J Oral Maxillofac Surg 1996;54(1):45-53; discussion 54.

[69] Turker N, Basa S, Vural G. Evaluation of osseous regeneration in alveolar distraction osteogenesis with histological and radiological aspects. J Oral Maxillofac Surg 2007;65(4):608-14.

[70] Perry M, Hodges N, Hallmon DW, Rees T, Opperman LA. Distraction osteogenesis versus autogenous onlay grafting. Part I: outcome of implant integration. Int J Oral Maxillofac Implants 2005;20(5):695-702.

[71] Uckan S, Oguz Y, Bayram B. Comparison of intraosseous and extraosseous alveolar distraction osteogenesis. J Oral Maxillofac Surg 2007;65(4):671-4.

[72] Bianchi A, Felice P, Lizio G, Marchetti C. Alveolar distraction osteogenesis versus inlay bone grafting in posterior mandibular atrophy: a prospective study. Oral Surg Oral Med Oral Pathol Oral Radiol Endod 2008;105(3):282-92.

[73] Jensen OT, Block M. Alveolar modification by distraction osteogenesis. Atlas Oral Maxillofac Surg Clin North Am 2008;16(2):185-214.

[74] Nocini PF, Albanese M, Buttura da Prato E, D'Agostino A. Vertical distraction osteogenesis of the mandible applied to an iliac crest graft: report of a case. Clin Oral Implants Res 2004;15(3):366-70.

[75] Dinse WE, Burnett RR. Anterior maxillary restoration using distraction osteogenesis and implants: a clinical report. J Prosthet Dent 2008;100(4):250-3.

[76] Gozneli R, Ozkan Y, Akalin ZF, Ozkan Y. Rehabilitation of maxillary anterior esthetics by alveolar distraction osteogenesis with immediate implant placement: a case report. Implant Dent;19(6):468-76.

[77] Lee HJ, Ahn MR, Sohn DS. Piezoelectric distraction osteogenesis in the atrophic maxillary anterior area: a case report. Implant Dent 2007;16(3):227-34.

[78] Penarrocha-Diago M, Gomez-Adrian MD, Garcia-Garcia A, Camacho-Alonso F, Rambla-Ferrer J. Vertical mandibular alveolar bone distraction and dental implant placement: a case report. J Oral Implantol 2006;32(3):137-41.

[79] Rachmiel A, Gutmacher Z, Blumenfeld I, Peled M, Laufer D. [Vertical alveolar ridge augmentation using distraction osteogenesis]. Refuat Hapeh Vehashinayim 2001;18(1):64-9, 78.

[80] Raghoebar GM, Liem RS, Vissink A. Vertical distraction of the severely resorbed edentulous mandible: a clinical, histological and electron microscopic study of 10 treated cases. Clin Oral Implants Res 2002;13(5):558-65.

[81] Yalcin S, Ordulu M, Emes Y, Gur H, Aktas I, Caniklioglu C. Alveolar distraction osteogenesis before placement of dental implants. Implant Dent 2006;15(1):48-52.

[82] Perdijk FB, Meijer GJ, Strijen PJ, Koole R. Complications in alveolar distraction osteogenesis of the atrophic mandible. Int J Oral Maxillofac Surg 2007;36(10):916-21.

[83] McAllister BS, Gaffaney TE. Distraction osteogenesis for vertical bone augmentation prior to oral implant reconstruction. Periodontol 2000 2003;33:54-66.

[84] Aikawa T, Iida S, Senoo H, Hori K, Namikawa M, Okura M, et al. Widening a narrow posterior mandibular alveolus following extirpation of a large cyst: a case treated with a titanium mesh-plate type distractor. Oral Surg Oral Med Oral Pathol Oral Radiol Endod 2008;106(5):e1-7.

[85] Bulut E, Muglali M, Celebi N, Bekcioglu B. Horizontal alveolar distraction of the mandibular canine regions for implant placement. J Craniofac Surg;21(3):830-2.

[86] Garcia-Garcia A, Somoza-Martin M, Gandara-Vila P, Saulacic N, Gandara-Rey JM. Horizontal alveolar distraction: a surgical technique with the transport segment pedicled to the mucoperiosteum. J Oral Maxillofac Surg 2004;62(11):1408-12.

[87] Laster Z, Rachmiel A, Jensen OT. Alveolar width distraction osteogenesis for early implant placement. J Oral Maxillofac Surg 2005;63(12):1724-30.

[88] Oda T, Suzuki H, Yokota M, Ueda M. Horizontal alveolar distraction of the narrow maxillary ridge for implant placement. J Oral Maxillofac Surg 2004;62(12):1530-4.

[89] Watzak G, Zechner W, Tepper G, Vasak C, Busenlechner D, Bernhart T. Clinical study of horizontal alveolar distraction with modified micro bone screws and subsequent implant placement. Clin Oral Implants Res 2006;17(6):723-9.

Advanced Oral and Maxillofacial Reconstruction

Chapter 4

Microsurgical Reconstruction of Maxillary Defects

Shahram Nazerani

Additional information is available at the end of the chapter

1. Introduction

The maxilla is the functional and esthetic keystone of the midface, forming part of each of the key midfacial elements; these are the orbits, the zygomatico-maxillary complex, the nasal unit, and the stomatognathic complex. Maxillary reconstruction is a challenging endeavor in functional and esthetic restoration. Given its central location in the midface and its contributions to the midface, maxillary defects are inherently complex because they generally involve more than one midfacial component. Maxillary defects are composite in nature, and they often require skin coverage, bony support, and mucosal lining for reconstruction. Reconstruction of maxillary defects secondary to warfare, trauma, ablative tumor surgery, or congenital deformities must meet the following goals namely: (1) obliteration of the defect; (2) restoration of essential functions such as mastication and speech, (3) provision for adequate structural support to each of the midfacial units and (4) esthetic restoration of facial features. This chapter will discuss the anatomic considerations, the historical approaches to maxillary reconstruction as well as state-of-the-art techniques in use today.

2. Anatomy

Understanding the complex three-dimensional anatomy of the maxilla and its relationship to contiguous structures is critical to approaching reconstruction of the midface. Conceptually, the maxilla can be described as a geometric structure with six walls (a hexahedron, Figure 1).

The roof of the box is the floor of the orbit; the floor forms the anterior hard palate and alveolar ridge; the lateral walls form the lateral walls of the maxillary sinuses and are a part of the lacrimal system. The maxillary sinus, the largest of the paranasal sinuses, is contained within the central portion of the maxilla. Anteriorly it comprises the midface supporting the nose and anterior teeth. Overlying the posterior pterygoid region of the maxilla is the cranial base.

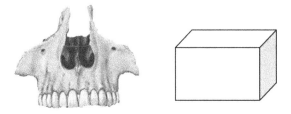

Figure 1. The maxilla and the schematic metaphor of a hexahedron.

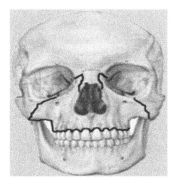

Figure 2. The maxilla with its surrounding bony structures.

The maxilla provides structural support between the skull base and the occlusal plane, supports the globe, separates the oral and nasal cavities and resists the forces of mastication. [1]

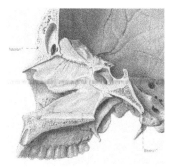

Figure 3. The maxilla with its projections create the bony foundation of the midface.

Finally, the overlying soft tissues, including the mimetic musculature of the midface, are supported by the maxilla and influence to a large extent one's unique facial appearance.

3. Historical procedures for maxillary reconstruction

Traditionally, reconstruction of large maxillary defects was accomplished by obturation of the defect with a prosthetic appliance. [2,3] Before the development of more sophisticated reconstructive techniques, prosthetic appliances were the only modality available to address the functional and esthetic requirements of such a complex defect. Both functional and esthetic results were far from optimal (Figure 4).

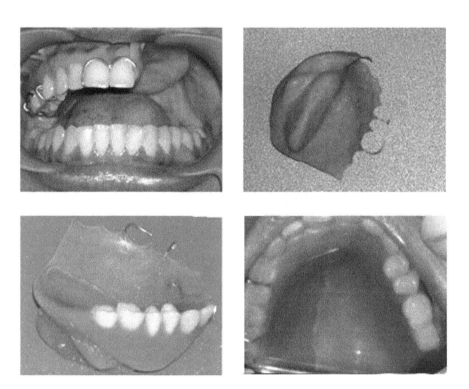

Figure 4. A hemi-maxillary obturator prosthesis.

Edgerton and Zovickian [4] reviewed early attempts at autogenous reconstruction of the maxilla and reported a palatal reconstruction technique using cervical flaps. These early reconstructive endeavors progressed from local flaps, such as forehead, upper lip, cheek, pharyngeal, turbinate, and tongue flaps, to tube flaps from the upper extremity, thorax, and abdomen. [5,6] Numerous other local flaps have been described for maxillary and palatal reconstruction. Generally, these have been useful for small defects or to augment other tissue-transfer techniques used to reconstruct larger defects. [7-17]

One of the earliest descriptions of a staged maxillary reconstruction with both soft tissue and bone was by Campbell in 1948. [18] He combined a temporalis muscle flap with a rotational palatal mucosal flap for soft-tissue reconstruction. An iliac bone graft was then placed in a second procedure; this was followed by the placement of a vestibular skin graft. The resulting reconstructed maxilla was capable of supporting a conventional maxillary denture.During the 1960s and 1970s, pedicled myocutaneous flaps were developed and replaced the more cumbersome tube flaps previously used in reconstructive surgery. However, these flaps tended to be quite bulky and were limited in their capacity to replicate the complexities of the resected maxillary structures. During the 1980s, a revolution in reconstructive surgery was brought about by the introduction of free tissue transfer techniques. These techniques have been widely applied in maxillary reconstruction, [18-25] and they have made possible the use of less bulky fascial or fasciocutaneous and osseous flaps. [26-36] Alongside the development of these tissue transfer techniques was the development of osseointegration pioneered by Branemark. [37-39] This technology, in combination with free tissue transfer, has made autogenous reconstruction of the maxilla and dentofacial rehabilitation possible. [40-45]

4. Classifying midfacial defects

Because of the disparate shapes and sizes of defects affecting the maxilla, the complex three-dimensional anatomy and the contiguous relationship of the maxilla to the surrounding structures, the broad category of maxillectomy constitute a wide spectrum of diverse defects. [46] Thus, a classification system to group this wide array of possible composite tissue defects was needed to facilitate clinical decision-making by outlining preferred reconstructive options and their common functional and esthetic sequelae. Attesting to both the variety and complexity of midfacial defects, numerous different classification schemes have been proposed. Based on a combined experience with 45 maxillectomies, Brown et al. developed a classification scheme allowing a very detailed description of 10 possible defects involving the palate; defects of the midface not involving the palate were excluded from the classification. [47] Unfortunately, the status of the orbital floor and zygoma, which play an important role in both the function and cosmesis of the midface, were not specifically addressed and specific recommendations for the reconstruction of each type was not given.

Wells and Luce proposed a classification system based on the extent of maxillary resections. [48] The schema allows the distinct classification of defects; however, proposed treatment focuses on the use of prosthetic obturators and/or the use of regional flaps rather than the specific use of microsurgical tissue transfer. In contrast, Yamamoto advocated the use of complex microsurgical procedures, specifically, the combined latissimus dorsi myocutaneous free flap with scapular bone based on the angular branch of the thoracodorsal artery and the rectus abdominis myocutaneous flap combined with costal cartilage based on the vascular connection between the eighth intercostal and deep epigastric vascular system. [49-50] Based on their 10-year experience with 38 maxillary reconstructions, they designed a complex reconstructive algorithm that ultimately culminates in nine different clinical scenarios based predominantly on the aforementioned vascularized, composite-tissue flaps. Futran and

Mendez presented an algorithm designed to depict options for midface reconstruction. Based on a thorough review of the literature, they classified defects as those involving the palate, the inferior maxilla, or the total maxilla with or without orbital exenteration. [46] Their algorithm was designed to delineate types of tissue required to reconstruct a particular defect, such as soft-tissue flaps or vascularized bone flaps rather than specific flap options. Spiro *et al.* proposed a relatively straightforward classification system that divides defects into three subtypes but does not specifically address the involvement of adjacent structures such as the orbit and zygoma. [51] based on a review of 108 patients, Davison *et al.* similarly divided patients into the two broad categories of "compete" or "partial" maxillectomy defects. [52] Although their group proposed a wide range of reconstructive techniques, the lack of a specific defect-oriented classification system outlining the remaining portion of the hard palate, dentition, orbit, and zygoma makes such an algorithm difficult to apply as a reconstructive guide. [53]

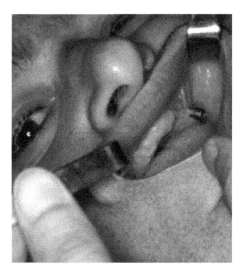

Figure 5. Maxillary atrophy after midface radiation for a small maxillary tumor 10 years back.

The same could be said for the classification proposed by Foster *et al.* [54] based on a single-surgeon series of 26 midfacial reconstructions; they classified defects into those involving soft-tissues and those involving bone. Bony midfacial defects were then subclassified into those involving more or less than half the palate. Triana *et al.* assessed 51 midfacial defects that had been treated with microvascular free-tissue transfer procedures. [55] The defects were classified as those seen after inferior partial maxillectomy, subtyped into the extent of palate lost and subdivided depending on the amount of malar bone and zygomatic arch lost. Okay *et al.* performed a retrospective review of 27 consecutive palatomaxillary reconstructions and designed a defect-oriented classification system designed to delineate the indication for prosthetic reconstruction, soft-tissue reconstruction, or vascularized bone-containing free flaps. [53] The authors concluded that the classification system does not address all factors required for decision-making. Although most of these classification systems allow for accurate descriptions of anatomical defects, many do not provide a clear algorithm for flap selection based on defect category. Others do not provide a comprehensive system for classifying defects of the midface that includes important structures such as the orbit or zygoma. One of the newer classifications has been proposed by McCarthy *et al.*56 They classify the maxillary defect of oncologic surgery origin into five distinct types; it is a rather straightforward classification but there are some deficiencies in this classification i.e. maxillary atrophy after radiation therapy (Figure 5,6).

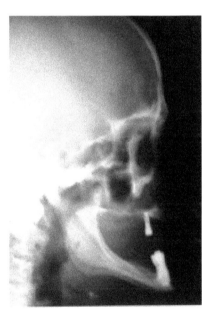

Figure 6. Lateral skull x ray showing the extent of atrophy of the mandible and maxilla.

An all inclusive classification is yet to be found; but as a rule of thumb maxillary reconstruction can be divided into three groups :

a.   *Upper maxilla* which needs space filling or bulky flaps

b.   *Lowermaxillaoralveolarridge* for which the prefabricated bone flaps are the best solution C: *Combined or total maxillary defects* in this group a single flap addressing both the problems is yet to be found.

The McCarthy classification is as follows:

4.1. Type l: Limited maxillectomy

Type l defects include resection of one or two walls of the maxilla, excluding the palate. In most cases, the anterior wall is partially removed with either the medial wall and/or, occasionally, the orbital rim. In addition, these resections commonly involve the overlying cheek and can extend onto the lips, nose, or eyelids. Thus, type l or limited maxillectomy defects usually require a significant amount of skin for resurfacing with minimal associated bone volume (Figure 7).

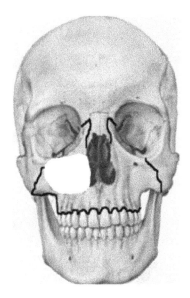

Figure 7. Type I defect of the right hemi-maxilla with the alveolar ridge intact.

4.1.1. Treatment

The radial forearm fasciocutaneous flap provides good external skin coverage and minimal bulk in this setting. Multiple skin islands can be designed and de-epithelialized when needed to wrap around bone grafts or supply nasal lining. If critical segments of bone are missing, such as the orbital rim or the anterior floor of the orbit, nonvascularized bone grafts can provide the needed support. Other flap options, depending on the amount of soft-tissue bulk required, include the lateral arm flap, anterolateral thigh flap, [57] and scapula flap. [58]

4.2. Type ll: Subtotal maxillectomy

Type ll defects include resection of the maxillary arch, hard palate, and anterior and lateral walls (five walls) with preservation of the orbital floor (Figure 8).

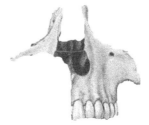

Figure 8. Type II defect, the alveolar ridge is removed but the floor of orbit is intact.

All type II defects involving more than 50 percent of the transverse palate require flaps that provide a substantial surface area with which to reline the nasal floor and palatal roof, and bone for structural support. [59-61] Similarly, in patients who do not have sufficient retentive surfaces and/or teeth to support a conventional prosthesis, vascularized bone-containing free flap reconstruction is indicated.

4.2.1. Treatment

The associated bulk provided by the skin and soft tissues is a significant disadvantage to using the fibula osteocutaneous flap, therefore we recommend the use of the prelaminated fibula free flap for the reconstruction of these defects (Figures 9-15).62

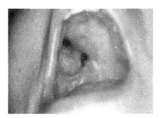

Figure 9. A defect created after a maxillary tumor with alveolar ridge loss (two years after surgery).

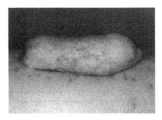

Figure 10. The prelaminated fibula created and matured on the leg.

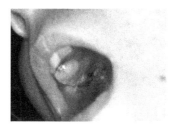

Figure 11. The flap has been transferred and the defect reconstructed.

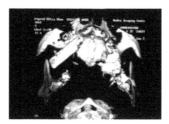

Figure 12. Axial CT scan showing the fibula in place.

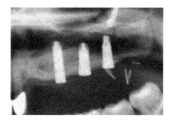

Figure 13. The x-ray after implant fixture insertion.

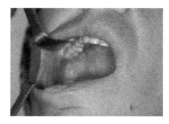

Figure 14. The fixed prosthesis in place.

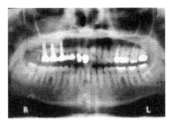

Figure 15. The panoramic view of the implant and the prelaminated fibula in place two years after surgery.

Various other donor sites have also been used to reconstruct these defects. Schliephake used a fasciocutaneous forearm flap followed by secondary bone grafting in two patients and reported that secondary nonvascularized bone grafting increases the risk of infection and is therefore not recommended. [63]

Use of the iliac crest free flap harvested with the internal oblique muscle has been reported by others. Iliac bone is plentiful and can provide a suitable bed for osseointegrated implants; however, its disadvantages include its short vascular pedicle and the potential for significant donor-site morbidity following its harvest. [58]

4.3. Type lll: Total maxillectomy

Type lll defects include resection of all six walls of the maxilla. These total maxillectomy defects are further subdivided into type lll a defects, where the orbital contents are preserved; and type lll b defects, where the orbital contents are exenterated.

4.3.1. Type llla

Reconstruction after total maxillectomy with preservation of the orbital contents is technically more challenging than maxillectomy with orbital exenteration. In this setting, reconstruction must: (1) provide support to the orbital contents, (2) obliterate any communication between the orbit and nasopharynx, and (3) reconstruct the palatal surface. When the orbital floor has been resected, support needs to be restored to the orbital contents; otherwise, the globe will prolapse downward, causing severe vertical dystopia with significant diplopia (Figure 16).

A variety of methods have been advocated to provide orbital support, including nonvascularized and vascularized bone grafts, alloplastic substitutes, and soft-tissue "slings." [64-65] we strongly advocate the use of **nonvascularized bone grafts** to support the orbital contents. By contrast, the use of alloplastic substitutes in defects that potentially expose it to the oronasal cavity increase the opportunity for periprosthetic infection. The volume of a soft-tissue flap may change over time [66] secondary to muscle atrophy, scar contracture, or changes in nutritional status. In this setting, even minor changes in volume can translate into significant changes in the vertical position of the soft-tissue sling and consequently the volume of the orbital cavity.

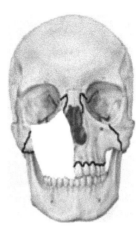

Figure 16. The defect created schematically shown; the floor of the orbit is intact.

By using the **rectus abdominis free flap** in combination with nonvascularized bone grafts, reconstruction of a three-dimensional defect is facilitated because the bone, skin, and soft-tissue components may be inset into their desired positions without compromising the microvascular aspect of the reconstruction. In addition, the rectus abdominis can be harvested easily during the resection and the pedicle can be extended up to 19 cm to reach the neck vessels.

Alternatively, the **temporalis flap** can be used to cover bone. Using this approach, however, requires the subsequent use of a palatal obturator; thus, the temporalis muscle flap is indicated primarily in older patients who are not candidates for free-tissue transfer. It is also useful for the patient who has an intact palate and preserved orbital contents (usually ethmoidal tumor resections), where access for free flap vessels is exceedingly difficult and muscle coverage is still needed to cover orbital bone grafts. [67] We however, support the use of vascularized bone flaps in this setting. The osteocutaneous free flap most frequently described for reconstruction of the maxillary region are the scapula, fibula, and radius. Each donor site has its own advantages and disadvantages.

The **osteocutaneous radial forearm flap** has been used for simultaneous reconstruction of the infraorbital margin and external skin in the midface. [68] Unfortunately, the volume of tissue transferred is rarely enough to obliterate the maxillary cavity completely, and palatal defects must be obturated with a prosthesis. [69]

Others have advocated the use of the **subscapular flap** to reconstruct defects caused by total maxillectomy with orbital preservation. Replacement of the alveolar arch inferiorly with the lateral scapular bone and the orbital floor and rim with the scapular tip has been described. [70] Schliephake reported difficulty however, in tailoring the scapular bone over the malar prominence, infraorbital rim, and maxillary wall at the same time that the lateral border of the scapula was to be positioned for placement of implants at the alveolar crest. [63] Yamamoto *et al.* have similarly reported using the scapular bone in conjunction with costal cartilage for reconstruction of all the maxillary buttresses in extended midfacial defects. [49]

Several authors have described the use of **free fibula osteocutaneous flaps** to reconstruct combined maxillary and mandible defects. [71] we think that the prefabricated fibula can address the alveolar ridge and the palate but cannot reconstruct both the mandible and maxilla in one setting and also the prefabricated fibula cannot act as a space filling flap for upper maxillary defects (Figure 17,18).

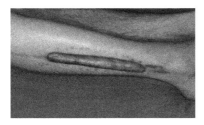

Figure 17. The matured fibula ready for transfer.

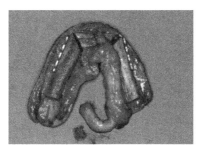

Figure 18. The "on table" preparation of the fibula has been done, the complete maxillary arch is created, the amount of soft tissue can only cover the palatal defect

However, Futran *et al.* found that as the need for reconstruction of the zygomatic complex, infraorbital rim, and the floor increased, the fibula flap was limited in its ability to restore the entire maxillary form. [67] In addition, it was difficult to osteotomize and orient the bone to restore both the palate and the infraorbital area. Even with the harvest of additional soleus muscle bulk, it was difficult to rotate the skin paddle to resurface the palate and provide zygomatic and infraorbital contour. Based on this experience, their group concluded that when orbitozygomatic support is the primary objective, use of the fibular free flap is not advocated.

Brown presented three cases of reconstruction with the **iliac crest myo-osseous flap** with favorable functional results. [47] A "block" of iliac bone was used to restore alveolus, zygomatic prominence, and orbital rim with success. Genden *et al.* Described use of the iliac crest–

internal oblique osteomusculocutaneous free flap in six patients, four of whom had type IIIa defects. [72] The iliac crest was fashioned to recreate the inferior orbital rim; the internal oblique muscle was used to reline the palate and resurface the ipsilateral lateral nasal wall. Based on their report, all four patients achieved facial symmetry and underwent placement of osseointegrated implants. Others have discouraged the use of this flap however, because of its potentially excessive bulk, limited soft-tissue mobility in relationship to the bone and short pedicle length. [70-73]

4.3.2. Type IIIb

Patients with type IIIb defects undergo resection of the entire maxilla in addition to exenteration of the orbit (also known as the extended maxillectomy). These defects are extensive and have both large-volume and large–surface area requirements. The palate needs to be closed; the medial wall of the maxilla often needs to be restored to maintain an adequate airway; and the often extensive external defect, which can involve the eyelids, cheek, and occasionally the lip, need to be reconstructed. In addition, the anterior cranial base in the area of the sphenoid is often exposed and coverage of the brain becomes essential (Figure 19).

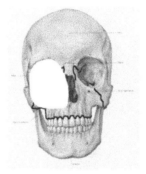

Figure 19. Type IIIb defect; the lower portion of maxilla is intact.

If the external skin of the cheek is intact, a rectus abdominis free flap with a skin island used to close the palate is a simple, straightforward solution. If the flap is not too bulky, a second skin island to restore the lateral nasal wall can be used. A third skin island can be used to provide closure of the external skin deficit if necessary.4 [73-75]

Shestak *et al*. successfully used the **latissimus dorsi flap** in three patients with type IIIb defects to fill the orbital cavity, seal the palate, and recontour the soft tissue of the face and cheek. [75] The latissimus dorsi was used because of its bulk, reliable anatomy, and ample pedicle length.

Palatal closure has its advantages and disadvantages in these reconstructions. If the palate is not closed (and muscle alone is used to cover the brain), the resultant massive intraoral defect requires a very large obturator, which can be difficult to support if there are no teeth left in the remaining maxilla. Palatal closure, although not ideal, makes sense because these patients can usually speak well and eat soft solids without dentures. Denture fitting can be difficult if the skin bulges downward and there are no teeth to fit the prosthesis. However, because these patients would have similar difficulties with an open palate and function well even without a denture when closed, we feel that the palatal closure is generally advisable.

We do not attempt to reconstruct bony deficits in these patients because of the extensive nature of the defects. Bone-containing free flaps do not have the same versatility with regard to providing intraoral and extraoral lining and soft-tissue bulk and are therefore not generally indicated for the massive type lllb resections.

4.4. Type lV: Orbitomaxillectomy

Type lV or orbitomaxillectomy defects include five walls of the maxilla and the orbital contents, leaving the dura and brain exposed. The palate is usually left intact with these resections. Reconstructive objectives include the provision of adequate soft tissue and the resurfacing of external skin defects where necessary. Thus, a flap that provides a medium volume of soft tissue and has the potential to cover a medium/large surface area with one or more skin islands is required (Figure 20).

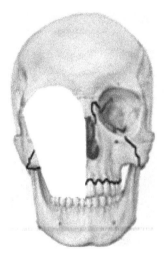

Figure 20. The complete defect with orbit involved.

The rectus abdominis flap can meet these requirements. These are conceptually simple reconstructive procedures, but the principal challenge is technical; one needs to anastomose the flap to a donor vessel in the neck, as temporal and facial vessels are usually resected or are unreliable. Dissection of the rectus pedicle extends the length up to 20 cm. A superficial tunnel in the face-lift plane allows transfer of the vessels; or, if the maxillary tubercle is resected, access can be gained by a parapharyngeal approach medial to the mandible. Maintaining the nasal airway is often the most difficult problem in these patients; thus, a second skin island to address lateral nasal wall reconstruction is helpful. [76]

4.5. Reconstruction with vascularized autogenous tissue

Advances in tissue transfer techniques have made sophisticated reconstruction with autogenous tissues possible. In the past, it was thought that autogenous reconstruction after tumor surgery would interfere with examination for residual or recurrent disease. Advances in diagnostic techniques such as computerized tomography, magnetic resonance imaging, and endoscopy now enable the surgeon to evaluate the resection bed without direct inspection. [77-80] With the numerous free and pedicled flaps and the adjunctive modalities, such as enteral feeding tubes, tracheostomy, and osseointegrated dental prostheses now available to the reconstructive surgeon, many of the technical difficulties related to autogenous reconstruction can be circumvented, both in the perioperative period and over the long term.

The idea of "one wound one scar" has drastically altered our reconstructive approaches. Local flaps in extensive defects only make a defect a "larger" defect and a "larger scar" ensues and in extensive maxillary defects "new" tissue must be brought into the wound and enlarging the scar by local or adjacent flaps is not advisable. The free or prefabricated flaps are not the "last ditch measures" and they must be considered as the first line of treatment in these complex midfacial defects (Figure 21,22).

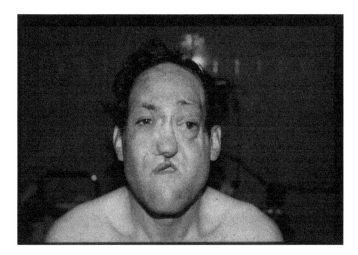

Figure 21. Frontal view, note the amount of forehead and upper lip scar.

Figures 21 shows a war-wounded veteran after 25 operations by world famous surgeons; the midface defect has been treated by local flaps, the maxillary defect remains and maxillary nonvascularized bone grafts, have all resorbed, the face and forehead are scarred.

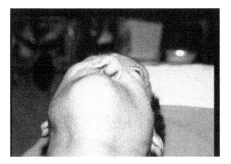

Figure 22. The maxillary defect from below.

5. State of the art procedures: Flap prefabrication and prelamination

Flap prefabrication is a term that was first introduced and later clinically applied by Shen in the early 1980s.81-82 Flap prefabrication and prelamination are two closely related concepts. Clinical applications of flap prefabrication and prelamination are relatively new to the field of reconstructive plastic surgery. Although the two terms are often used interchangeably in the literature, they are two distinctly different techniques. Understanding their differences is helpful in planning the reconstructive strategy. They are primarily used in reconstructing complex defects where conventional techniques are not indicated.

5.1. Flap prefabrication

Flap prefabrication starts with introduction of a vascular pedicle to a desired donor tissue that on its own does not possess an axial blood supply. After a period of neovascularization of at least 8 weeks, this donor tissue can then be transferred to the recipient defect based on the newly acquired axial vasculature (Figure 23).

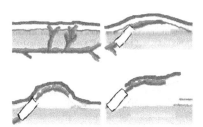

Figure 23. Flap prefabrication stages; vascular pedicle transferred under the skin paddle and the pedicle wrapped by either PTFE or silicone 62 and sometimes a tissue expander is inserted for expansion; the flap after proper expansion is transferred as a free or island flap.

Cartilage and bone can be incorporated into these flaps but they are mostly suitable for ear and nose reconstruction and for maxillary or mandibular reconstructions the prelamination method is the better choice. Flap prelamination, begins with building a three-dimensional structure on a reliable vascular bed. This composite structure, once matured in approximately 6-8 weeks can then be transferred to the recipient defect.

5.2. Flap prelamination

Flap prelamination is a term first coined by Pribaz and Fine in 1994. [83] The definition of "lamination" means bonding of thin sheets together to give a multilayered construction. In reconstructive surgery, the term "flap prelamination" has been used to describe a process of two or more stages for constructing a complex three-dimensional structure. The first stage involves adding different layers to an existing axial vascular territory as composite grafts, allowing time for the tissues to mature before being transferred (Figure 24-26).

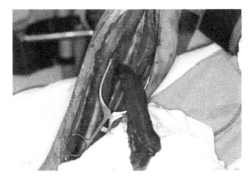

Figure 24. The fibula with the muscle cuff has been dissected and is attached to the leg via its vascular pedicle.

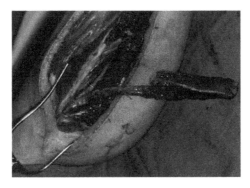

Figure 25. The pedicle has been prepared up to the trifurcation of the artery.

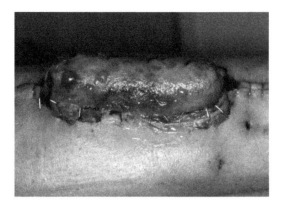

Figure 26. The pedicle is wrapped in silicone sheet and the bone flap is fixed to the leg surface and covered by a split-thickness skin graft, (postoperative day 10).

An intermediate stage may be needed to further modify the flap, such as thinning, delaying, or adding additional tissue. [84] At the next stage, when the remote composite flap is completed, it is transferred to the defect based on the original axial blood supply. As with any composite graft, these added layers have to be sufficiently thin or small for them to take. The rationale for prelaminating those layers at a different site before transfer results from the belief that this offers the best chance for the prelaminating layers to heal, stabilize, and assume their expected structures and positions if the construction is performed in a reliable vascular bed at a less conspicuous site instead of in situ, where local complicating factors can be numerous. This is particularly important for reconstruction of functional units that need to be transferred to complex local environments, where structural leaks may cause grave complications (e.g., neourethra in the perineum and neoesophagus in the mediastinum).

5.3. Flap maturation

Because the blood supply is not manipulated, the time for a prelaminated flap to mature is shorter than for a prefabricated flap, [85] usually between 4 and 6 weeks. Intuitively, this makes sense because it represents a similar amount of time for any composite graft to fully take, whereas in a prefabricated flap, neovascularization needs to take place over a much larger and sometimes thicker dimension of tissue. Intermediate manipulation may be required to obtain a thinner flap or to delay an extended portion of a flap or to add additional graft material (Figure 27).

5.4. Flap transfer

Because the layering of structures takes place in an established vascular territory, venous congestion is usually not a problem in a prelaminated flap as it is often in a prefabricated flap. However, all flaps, including prelaminated flaps, become edematous after transfer, and there is increased scarring at each tissue healing interface. In attempting to reconstruct complex

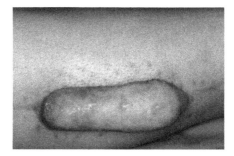

Figure 27. Postoperative week 8,the flap is completely matured and ready for transfer

three-dimensional structures, the multiple layers with scarring and contractile forces at each interface can result in distortion and loss of contour of the flap. Because of this, the initial result is often suboptimal, and generally several revisions are necessary. This occurs especially in the face, where prelamination is used for reconstruction of central facial features, such as the nose and surrounding tissues. Once the prelaminated flap is healed in place and a stable foundation has been obtained, the external part can be de-epithelialized and covered with local advancement flaps or, in the case of nostril reconstruction, with a forehead flap for final esthetic reconstruction (Figure 28,29).

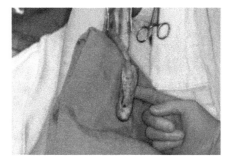

Figure 28. The flap has been dissected free from the leg and hangs on the pedicle which is wrapped in silicone, the dissection of the pedicle is fascilitated by the silicone sheet

6. Osseointegration techniques

The development of osseointegrated implants has revolutionized the approach to the dental rehabilitation of patients requiring maxillary reconstruction. The work of Branemark [86] and others has resulted in the development of the materials and techniques necessary to provide predictable and reliable implants that can be completely incorporated into grafted bone and

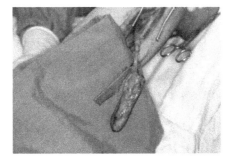

Figure 29. The silicone sheet is removed and the flap is ready for transfer.

support a fixed and stable dental prosthesis. [87-94] The use of osseointegrated implants in conjunction with free tissue transfer represents state-of-the-art reconstruction of large maxillary defects. The use of osseointegrated implants for dental rehabilitation has previously been much more extensively discussed in the context of mandibular reconstruction than that of maxillary reconstruction. [95] Some fundamental concepts of functional dental restoration with prosthetics should be understood. The reconstruction should provide for retention, support, and stabilization of the denture. Retention involves preventing the displacement of the prosthesis from the denture-bearing surface. Support implies that masticatory forces should not cause the prosthesis to impact vertically against the soft tissue of the load-bearing surface. Stabilization refers to the prevention of excessive lateral movement of the prosthesis. Dentures may be implant-borne, in which case the osseointegrated implants completely retain, support, and stabilize the prosthesis, or implant-retained, in which case the support and stabilization functions are shared by the denture-bearing surface and the retention of the prosthesis is completely dependent on the osseointegrated implants. Dentures that do not require osseointegrated implants are tissue-borne and tooth-supported, relying on the native tissues for retention and stabilization. [96]

Tissue-borne prostheses generally cannot be used in extensive maxillary defects because of insufficient residual palatal and alveolar tissues to provide support and retention. Funk *et al.* [96] defined such defects as those involving more than two-thirds of the maxillary arch. These defects typically require surgical reconstruction of the maxillary arch to provide neoalveolar bone of adequate thickness (approximately 10 mm) to accommodate osseointegrated implants, support a denture, and prevent its movement during mastication (Figure 30-34).

Bony reconstruction of the maxillary arch allows placement of the osseointegrated implants axial to the occlusal forces, a key factor for successful implant function. [96] Osseointegrated implants may be placed at the time of the reconstruction or secondarily, 6 to 8 weeks later. [96] Three to 8 months after placement, the osseointegrated implants are uncovered and prepared for final prosthetic reconstruction by a prosthodontist. [95]

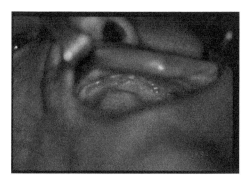

Figure 30. The maxillary defect after shrapnel injury.

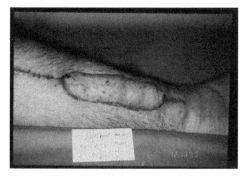

Figure 31. The matured fibula ready for transfer.

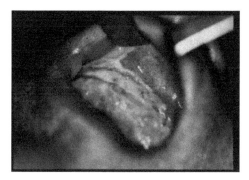

Figure 32. The fibula in place six months after surgery, please note the dark color of the grafted skin

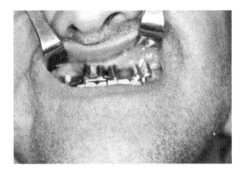

Figure 33. The patient ten years after surgery with implant in place, the skin graft has completely transformed into mucosa and is glistening and has the color of mucosa.

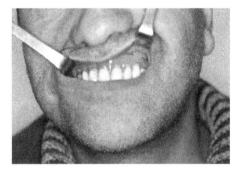

Figure 34. The dentures in place, ten year postoperatively.

The use of free tissue transfer techniques in combination with osseointegrated implants for maxillary reconstruction has been reported by various authors. [97] Holle *et al.* [98] described a two-stage procedure for the reconstruction of maxillectomy defects. Initially, an osseous flap was created from the lateral border of the scapula; it incorporated osseointegrated implants, was covered with skin grafts, and was protected with a PTFE membrane. Three months later, the flap was harvested and transferred to the face using a microsurgical technique. This procedure successfully restored facial contour and allowed full dental rehabilitation. Funk *et al.* [59] used free scapular osseocutaneous flaps with primary or secondary osseointegrated implants for large palatomaxillary defects in three patients. These patients all underwent successful dental rehabilitation, with 94 percent stability of the implants at an average of 18 months after the completion of rehabilitation. Nakayama *et al.* [99] reconstructed a bilateral maxillectomy defect with a free fibula osseocutaneous flap combined with osseointegrated implants. Igawa *et al.* [100] recently reported the use of a prefabricated iliac crest free flap, which was secondarily vascularized by a rectus abdominis muscle flap and covered by split-thickness skin graft, with the secondary placement of osseointegrated implants for functional alveolar ridge reconstruction after hemimaxillectomy.

7. Summary

Maxillary defects are one of the most challenging problems facing the reconstructive surgeon. Microsurgical tissue transfers evolved from the groin flap transfer to the complicated flap prefabrication and prelamination approaches to difficult reconstructive needs. These sophisticated techniques are distinctively different and yet can be perfectly complementary. Prelamination can add virtually anything to where there is a good axial blood supply, and prefabrication can bring an axial blood supply to almost anywhere in the body. The two techniques can even be combined when certain complex reconstructive needs are present. Prefabrication and prelamination can also serve as a conduit through which products of tissue engineering and embryonic stem cell technologies can be applied to the reconstruction of head and neck defects. Tissues synthesized in vitro with better structural, color, texture, and functional match can be prelaminated to a site that has already been prefabricated. Prefabrication of a bioabsorbable matrix system can create a well perfused scaffold to which more and larger subunits can be prelaminated.

As our understanding of the techniques evolves, the breadth of their usage will also expand. These techniques will continue to be useful to help solve many difficult problems that baffle even the very best reconstructive surgeons, and the potential for these techniques may be used to bring tissue engineering from the laboratory to clinical reality. Lastly, as progress is made in transplant pharmacology, the immunologic barrier to feasible composite tissue allograft transplantation may be overcome. This represents the beginning of a new era in reconstructive surgery.

Author details

Shahram Nazerani[1,2]

1 Associate Professor of Surgery, Firouzgar Hospital, Teheran, Iran

2 Tehran University of Medical Sciences, Tehran, Iran

References

[1] Schendel, S. A., and Delaire, J. Facial Muscles: Form, Function, and Reconstruction in Dentofacial Deformities. In W. H. Bell (Ed.), *Surgical Correction of Dentofacial Deformities*, Vol. 3. Philadelphia: Saunders, 1985.

[2] Hammond, J. Dental care of edentulous patients after resection of maxilla. *Br. Dent. J.* 120: 591, 1966.

[3] Curtis, T. A., and Beumer, J. Restoration of Acquired Hard Palate Defects: Etiology, Disability, and Rehabilitation. In J. Beumer, T. A. Curtis, and M. T. Marunick (Eds.), *Maxillofacial Rehabilitation: Prosthodontic and Surgical Considerations.* St. Louis: Ishiyaku EuroAmerica, 1996.

[4] Edgerton, M. T., Jr., and Zovickian, A. Reconstruction of major defects of the palate. *Plast. Reconstr. Surg.* 17: 105, 1956.

[5] Converse, J. M. Early and late treatment of gunshot wounds of the jaw in French battle casualties in North Africa and Italy. *J. Oral Surg.* 3: 112, 1945.

[6] Miller, T. A. The Tagliacozzi flap as a method of nasal and palatal reconstruction. *Plast. Reconstr. Surg.* 76: 870, 1985.

[7] Miller, T. A. The Tagliacozzi flap as a method of nasal and palatal reconstruction. *Plast. Reconstr. Surg.* 76: 870, 1985.

[8] Elliott, R. A., Jr. Use of nasolabial skin flap to cover intraoral defects. *Plast. Reconstr. Surg.* 58: 201, 1976.

[9] Chambers, R. G., Jaques, D. A., and Mahoney, W. D. Tongue flaps for intraoral reconstruction. *Am. J. Surg.* 118: 783, 1969.

[10] Jackson, I. T. *Local Flaps in Head and Neck Reconstruction.* St. Louis: Mosby, 1985.

[11] Niederdellmann, H., Munker, G., and Lange, G. Reconstruction of a defect of the orbital floor with a rotated flap from the nasal wall: A case report. *J. Maxillofac. Surg.* 2: 153, 1974.

[12] Crow, M. L., and Crow, F. J. Resurfacing large cheek defects with rotation flaps from the neck. *Plast. Reconstr. Surg.* 58: 196, 1976.

[13] Edgerton, M. T., and DeVito, R. V. Closure of palatal defects by means of a hinged nasal septum flap. *Plast. Reconstr. Surg.* 31: 537, 1963.

[14] Becker, D. W., Jr. A cervicopectoral rotation flap for cheek coverage. *Plast. Reconstr. Surg.* 61: 868, 1978.

[15] Guerrerosantos, J., and Altamirano, J. T. The use of lingual flaps in repair of fistulas of the hard palate. *Plast. Reconstr. Surg.* 38: 123, 1966.

[16] Wallace, A. F. Esser's skin flap for closing large palatal fistulae. *Br. J. Plast. Surg.* 19: 322, 1966.

[17] Komisar, A., and Lawson, W. A compendium of intraoral flaps. *Head Neck Surg.* 8: 91, 1985.

[18] Campbell, H. H. Reconstruction of the left maxilla. *Plast. Reconstr. Surg.* 3: 66, 1948.

[19] Baker, S. R. Closure of large orbito-maxillary defects with free latissimus dorsi myo-cutaneous flaps. *Head Neck Surg.* 6: 828, 1984.

[20] Matloub, H. S., Larson, D. L., Kuhn, J. C., *et al.* Lateral arm free flap in oral cavity reconstruction: A functional evaluation. *Head Neck Surg.* 11: 205, 1989.

[21] Matloub, H. S., Sanger, J. R., and Godina, M. Lateral Arm Neurosensory Flap. In H. B. Williams (Ed.), *Transactions of the 8th International Congress on Plastic and Reconstructive Surgery.* Montreal: International Plastic and Reconstructive Surgery, 1983. P. 125.

[22] Jones, N. F., Hardesty, R. A., Swartz, W. M., *et al.* Extensive and complex defects of the scalp, middle third of the face, and palate: The role of microsurgical reconstruction. *Plast. Reconstr. Surg.* 82: 937, 1988.

[23] Inoue, T., Harashina, T., Asanami, S., and Fujino, T. Reconstruction of the hard palate using free iliac bone covered with jejunal flap. *Br. J. Plast. Surg.* 41: 143, 1988.

[24] Panje, W. R., Krause, C. J., Bardach, J., and Baker, S. R. Reconstruction of intraoral defects with the free groin flap. *Arch. Otolaryngol.* 103: 78, 1977.

[25] Vaughan, E. D. The radial forearm free flap in orofacial reconstruction: Personal experience in 120 consecutive cases. *J. Craniomaxillofac. Surg.* 18: 2, 1990.

[26] Vuillemin, T., Raveh, J., and Ramon, Y. Reconstruction of the maxilla with bone grafts supported by the buccal fat pad. *J. Oral Maxillofac. Surg.* 46: 100, 1988.

[27] Kruger, E. Reconstruction of bone and soft tissue in extensive facial defects. *J. Oral Maxillofac. Surg.* 40: 714, 1982.

[28] McCarthy, J. G., and Zide, B. M. The spectrum of calvarial bone grafting: Introduction of the vascularized calvarial bone flap. *Plast. Reconstr. Surg.* 74: 10, 1984.

[29] Cutting, C. B., McCarthy, J. G., and Berenstein, A. Blood supply of the upper craniofacial skeleton: The search for composite calvarial bone flaps. *Plast. Reconstr. Surg.* 74: 603, 1984.

[30] Yaremchuk, M. J. Vascularized bone grafts for maxillofacial reconstruction. *Clin. Plast. Surg.* 16: 29, 1989.

[31] Antonyshyn, O., Gruss, J. S., and Birt, B. D. Versatility of temporal muscle and fascial flaps. *Br. J. Plast. Surg.* 41: 118, 1988.

[32] Serafin, D., Riefkohl, R., Thomas, I., and Georgiade, N. G. Vascularized rib periosteal and osteocutaneous reconstruction of the maxilla and mandible: An assessment. *Plast. Reconstr. Surg.* 66: 718, 1980.

[33] Lind, M. G., Arnander, C., Gylbert, L., *et al.* Reconstruction in the head and neck regions with free radial forearm flaps and split-rib bone grafts. *Am. J. Surg.* 154: 459, 1987.

[34] MacLeod, A. M., Morrison, W. A., McCann, J. J., *et al.* The free radial forearm flap with and without bone for closure of large palatal fistulae. *Br. J. Plast. Surg.* 40: 391, 1987.

[35] Conley, J., and Patow, C. Cranio Osseo-Myofascial Flaps. In J. J. Conley (Ed.), *Flaps in Head and Neck Surgery*. New York: Thieme Medical Publishing, 1989.

[36] Casanova, R., Cavalcante, D., Grotting, J. C., Vasconez, L. O., and Psillakis, J. M. Anatomic basis for vascularized outer table calvarial bone flaps. *Plast. Reconstr. Surg.* 78: 300, 1986.

[37] Branemark, P. I. Osseointegration and its experimental background. *J. Prosthet. Dent.* 50: 399, 1983.

[38] Jackson, I. T., Tolman, D. E., Desjardins, R. P., and Branemark, P. I. A new method for fixation of external prostheses. *Plast. Reconstr. Surg.* 77: 668, 1986.

[39] Tjellstrom, A., and Jacobsson, M. The Bone Anchored Maxillofacial Prosthesis. In T. Albrektson and G. Zarb (Eds.), *The Branemark Osseointegrated Implant*. Chicago: Quintessence Publishing, 1989.

[40] Holle, J., Vinzenz, K., Wuringer, E., *et al.* The prefabricated combined scapula flap for bony and soft-tissue reconstruction in maxillofacial defects: A new method. *Plast. Reconstr. Surg.* 98: 542, 1996.

[41] Li, K. K., Stephens, W. L., and Gliklich, R. Reconstruction of the severely atrophic edentulous maxilla using Le Fort I osteotomy with simultaneous bone graft and implant placement. *J. Oral Maxillofac. Surg.* 54: 542, 1996.

[42] Schmelzeisen, R., Neukam, F. W., Shirota, T., *et al.* Postoperative function after implant insertion in vascularized bone grafts in maxilla and mandible. *Plast. Reconstr. Surg.* 97: 719, 1996.

[43] Nakayama, B., Matsuura, H., Ishihara, O., *et al.* Functional reconstruction of a bilateral maxillectomy defect using a fibula osteocutaneous flap with osseointegrated implants. *Plast. Reconstr. Surg.* 96: 1201, 1995.

[44] Arcuri, M. R. Titanium implants in maxillofacial reconstruction. *Otolaryngol. Clin. North Am.* 28: 351, 1995.

[45] Donovan, M. G., Dickerson, N. C., Hanson, L. J., and Gustafson, R. B. Maxillary and mandibular reconstruction using calvarial bone grafts and Branemark implants: A preliminary report. *J. Oral Maxillofac. Surg.* 52: 588, 1994.

[46] Futran ND, Mendez E. Developments in reconstruction of midface and maxilla. *Lancet Oncol.* 2006;7:249–258.

[47] Brown JS, Rogers SN, McNally DN, Boyle M. A modified classification for the maxillectomy defect. *Head Neck* 2000;22:17–26.

[48] Wells MD, Luce EA. Reconstruction of midfacial defects after surgical resection of malignancies. *Clin Plast Surg.* 1995;22:79–89.

[49] Yamamoto Y, Kawashima K, Sugihara T, Nohira K, Furuta Y, Fukuda S. Surgical management of maxillectomy defects based on the concept of buttress reconstruction. *Head Neck* 2004;26:247–256.

[50] Yamamoto Y. Mid-facial reconstruction after maxillectomy. *Int J Clin Oncol.* 2005;10:218–222.

[51] Spiro RH, Strong EW, Shah JP. Maxillectomy and its classification. *Head Neck* 1997;19:309–314.

[52] Davison SP, Sherris DA, Meland NB. An algorithm for maxillectomy defect reconstruction. *Laryngoscope* 1998;108:215–219.

[53] Okay DJ, Genden E, Buchbinder D, Urken M. Prosthodontic guidelines for surgical reconstruction of the maxilla: A classification system of defects. *J Prosthet Dent.* 2001;86:352–363.

[54] Foster RD, Anthony JP, Singer MI, Kaplan MJ, Pogrel MA, Mathes SJ. Microsurgical reconstruction of the midface. *Arch Surg.* 1996;131:960–965; discussion 965–966.

[55] Triana RJ Jr, Uglesic V, Virag M, *et al.* Microvascular free flap reconstructive options in patients with partial and total maxillectomy defects. *Arch Facial Plast Surg.* 2000;2:91–101.

[56] McCarthy, Colleen M. M.D., M.S.; Cordeiro, Peter G. M.D. Microvascular Reconstruction of Oncologic Defects of the Midface, *Plastic & Reconstructive Surgery.* 2010 ;126 :6 ; 1947-1959

[57] Amin A, Rifaat M, Civantos F, Weed D, Abu-Sedira M, Bassiouny M. Free anterolateral thigh flap for reconstruction of major craniofacial defects. *J Reconstr Microsurg.* 2006;22:97–104.

[58] Archibald S, Jackson S, Thoma A. Paranasal sinus and midfacial reconstruction. *Clin Plast Surg.* 2005;32:309–325.

[59] Funk GF, Arcuri MR, Frodel JL Jr. Functional dental rehabilitation of massive palato-maxillary defects: Cases requiring free tissue transfer and osseointegrated implants. *Head Neck* 1998;20:38–51.

[60] Genden EM, Wallace DI, Okay D, Urken ML. Reconstruction of the hard palate using the radial forearm free flap: Indications and outcomes. *Head Neck* 2004;26:808–814.

[61] Cordeiro PG, Bacilious N, Schantz S, Spiro R. The radial forearm osteocutaneous "sandwich" free flap for reconstruction of the bilateral subtotal maxillectomy defect. *Ann Plast Surg.* 1998;40:397–402.

[62] Nazerani S, Behnia H, Motamedi MH . Experience with the prefabricated free fibula flap for reconstruction of maxillary and mandibular defects. J Oral Maxillofac Surg. 2008 Feb;66(2):260-4.

[63] .Schliephake H. Revascularized tissue transfer for the repair of complex midfacial defects in oncologic patients. *J Oral Maxillofac Surg.* 2000;58:1212–1218.

[64] Cinar C, Arslan H, Ogur S, Kilic A, Bingol UA, Yucel A. Free rectus abdominis myocutaneous flap with anterior rectus sheath to provide the orbital support in globe-sparing total maxillectomy. *J Craniofac Surg.* 2006;17:986–991.

[65] .Askar I, Oktay MF, Kilinc N. Use of radial forearm free flap with palmaris longus tendon in reconstruction of total maxillectomy with sparing of orbital contents. *J Craniofac Surg.* 2003;14:220–227.

[66] Sarukawa S, Okazaki M, Asato H, Koshima I. Volumetric changes in the transferred flap after anterior craniofacial reconstruction. *J Reconstr Microsurg.* 2006;22:499–505; discussion 506–507.

[67] Futran ND, Haller JR. Considerations for free-flap reconstruction of the hard palate. *Arch Otolaryngol Head Neck Surg.* 1999;125:665–669.

[68] McLoughlin PM, Gilhooly M, Phillips JG. Reconstruction of the infraorbital margin with a composite microvascular free flap. *Br J Oral Maxillofac Surg.* 1993;31:227–229.

[69] Chepeha DB, Moyer JS, Bradford CR, Prince ME, Marentette L, Teknos TN. Osseocutaneous radial forearm free tissue transfer for repair of complex midfacial defects. *Arch Otolaryngol Head Neck Surg.* 2005;131:513–517.

[70] Coleman JJ III. Osseous reconstruction of the midface and orbits. *Clin Plast Surg.* 1994;21:113–124.

[71] Taylan G, Yildirim S, Akoz T. Reconstruction of large orbital exenteration defects after resection of periorbital tumors of advanced stage. *J Reconstr Microsurg.* 2006;22:583–589.

[72] Genden EM, Wallace D, Buchbinder D, Okay D, Urken ML. Iliac crest internal oblique osteomusculocutaneous free flap reconstruction of the postablative palatomaxillary defect. *Arch Otolaryngol Head Neck Surg.* 2001;127:854–861.

[73] Cordeiro PG, Disa JJ. Challenges in midface reconstruction. *Semin Surg Oncol.* 2000;19:218–225.

[74] Taylan G, Yildirim S, Akoz T. Reconstruction of large orbital exenteration defects after resection of periorbital tumors of advanced stage. *J Reconstr Microsurg.* 2006;22:583–589.

[75] Shestak KC, Schusterman MA, Jones NF, Johnson JT. Immediate microvascular reconstruction of combined palatal and midfacial defects using soft tissue only. *Microsurgery* 1988;9:128–131.

[76] Cordeiro PG, Santamaria E. A classification system and algorithm for reconstruction of maxillectomy and midfacial defects. *Plast Reconstr Surg.* 2000;105:2331–2346; discussion

[77] Boyne, P. J., Christiansen, E. L., and Thompson, J. R. Advanced imaging of osseous maxillary clefts. *Radiol. Clin. North Am.* 31: 195, 1993.

[78] Metes, A., Hoffstein, V., Direnfeld, V., *et al.* Three-dimensional CT reconstruction and volume measurements of the pharyngeal airway before and after maxillofacial surgery in obstructive sleep apnea. *J. Otolaryngol.* 22: 261, 1993.

[79] Remonda, L., Schroth, G., Ozdoba, C., *et al.* Facial intraosseous arteriovenous malformations: CT and MR features. *J. Comput. Assist. Tomogr.* 19: 277, 1995.

[80] Bradrick, J. P., Smith, A. S., Ohman, J. C., and Indresano, A. T. Estimation of maxillary alveolar cleft volume by three-dimensional CT. *J. Comput. Assist. Tomogr.* 14: 994, 1990.

[81] Shen ZY. Vascular implantation into skin flap: Experimental study and clinical application. A preliminary report. *Plast Reconstr Surg.* 1981;68:404–410.

[82] Shen ZY. Microvascular transplantation of prefabricated free thigh flap (letter). *Plast Reconstr Surg.* 1982;69:568.

[83] Pribaz JJ, Fine NA. Prelamination: Defining the prefabricated flap. A case report and review. *Microsurgery* 1994;15:618–623.

[84] Walton RL, Burget GC, Beahm EK. Microsurgical reconstruction of the nasal lining. *Plast Reconstr Surg.* 2005;115:1813–1829.

[85] Pribaz JJ, Fine NA. Prefabricated and prelaminated flaps for head and neck reconstruction. *Clin Plast Surg.* 2001;28:261–272.

[86] Branemark, P. I. Osseointegration and its experimental background. *J. Prosthet. Dent.* 50: 399, 1983.

[87] Jackson, I. T., Tolman, D. E., Desjardins, R. P., and Branemark, P. I. A new method for fixation of external prostheses. *Plast. Reconstr. Surg.* 77: 668, 1986.

[88] Tjellstrom, A., and Jacobsson, M. The Bone Anchored Maxillofacial Prosthesis. In T. Albrektson and G. Zarb (Eds.), *The Branemark Osseointegrated Implant.* Chicago: Quintessence Publishing, 1989.

[89] Holle, J., Vinzenz, K., Wuringer, E., *et al.* The prefabricated combined scapula flap for bony and soft-tissue reconstruction in maxillofacial defects: A new method. *Plast. Reconstr. Surg.* 98: 542, 1996.

[90] Li, K. K., Stephens, W. L., and Gliklich, R. Reconstruction of the severely atrophic edentulous maxilla using Le Fort I osteotomy with simultaneous bone graft and implant placement. *J. Oral Maxillofac. Surg.* 54: 542, 1996.

[91] Schmelzeisen, R., Neukam, F. W., Shirota, T., *et al.* Postoperative function after implant insertion in vascularized bone grafts in maxilla and mandible. *Plast. Reconstr. Surg.* 97: 719, 1996.

[92] Nakayama, B., Matsuura, H., Ishihara, O., *et al.* Functional reconstruction of a bilateral maxillectomy defect using a fibula osteocutaneous flap with osseointegrated implants. *Plast. Reconstr. Surg.* 96: 1201, 1995.

[93] Arcuri, M. R. Titanium implants in maxillofacial reconstruction. *Otolaryngol. Clin. North Am.* 28: 351, 1995.

[94] Donovan, M. G., Dickerson, N. C., Hanson, L. J., and Gustafson, R. B. Maxillary and mandibular reconstruction using calvarial bone grafts and Branemark implants: A preliminary report. *J. Oral Maxillofac. Surg.* 52: 588, 1994.

[95] Urken, M. L., Buchbinder, D., Weinberg, H., *et al.* Primary placement of osseointegrated implants in microvascular mandibular reconstruction. *Otolaryngol. Head Neck Surg.* 101: 56, 1989.

[96] Funk, G. F., Arcuri, M. R., and Frodel, J. L., Jr. Functional dental rehabilitation of massive palatomaxillary defects: Cases requiring free tissue transfer and osseointegrated implants. *Head Neck* 20: 38, 1998.

[97] Schmelzeisen, R., Neukam, F. W., Shirota, T., *et al.* Postoperative function after implant insertion in vascularized bone grafts in maxilla and mandible. *Plast. Reconstr. Surg.* 97: 719, 1996.

[98] Holle, J., Vinzenz, K., Wuringer, E., *et al.* The prefabricated combined scapula flap for bony and soft-tissue reconstruction in maxillofacial defects: A new method. *Plast. Reconstr. Surg.* 98: 542, 1996.

[99] Nakayama, B., Matsuura, H., Ishihara, O., *et al.* Functional reconstruction of a bilateral maxillectomy defect using a fibula osteocutaneous flap with osseointegrated implants. *Plast. Reconstr. Surg.* 96: 1201, 1995.

[100] Igawa, H. H., Minakawa, H., and Sugihara, T. Functional alveolar ridge reconstruction with prefabricated iliac crest free flap and osseointegrated implants after hemimaxillectomy. *Plast. Reconstr. Surg.* 102: 2420, 1998.

Chapter 5

Reconstruction of Mandibular Defects

Maiolino Thomaz Fonseca Oliveira,
Flaviana Soares Rocha, Jonas Dantas Batista,
Sylvio Luiz Costa de Moraes and
Darceny Zanetta-Barbosa

Additional information is available at the end of the chapter

1. Introduction

Surgical reconstruction of mandibular bone defects is a routine procedure for rehabilitation of patients with deformities caused by trauma, infection or tumor resection. The mandible plays a major role in masticatory and phonetic functions, supporting the teeth and defining the contour of the lower third of the face. Therefore, mandibular discontinuity produces severe cosmetic and functional deformities, including loss of support for suprahyoid muscles and subsequent airway reduction. Reconstruction of these severe defects is mandatory for restoring the patient's quality of life. Surgical techniques have improved considerably in the last decade, but reconstruction of large bone defects of the mandible still pose a great challenge in maxillofacial rehabilitation. Several things can be done to optimize the surgery; the use of prototyping modeling for instance provides a better assessment of the bone defect and pre-contouring of the fixation plates, reducing operating time. The choice of the most suitable titanium plate system is critical to the success of the procedure. Mandibular defects with loss of continuity require more robust (load bearing) systems supporting mandibular function. Many studies consider the use of plates and screws temporary treatment due to the large number of complications such as fracture of plates and screws, plate exposure and infection. Thus, the use of grafts both in the first operation or in a two-stage procedure ensures a more predictable result.

Bone grafts are widely used in reconstructive surgery of the mandible. Incorporation of the bone graft restores continuity, shape, and strength of the jaw to near normal function. Installation of dental implants in the grafted areas is important to restore masticatory function and maintain bone graft volume. Autogenous bone is the best choice for major reconstructions due to lack of rejection, and the presence of viable osteogenic cells that increase bone formation and incorporation at the graft site. The use of a vascularized graft is a good choice because it increases the success of the treatment. However, this technique is not available in all medical centers. Autogenous free bone (non-vascularized) is still the most used graft, even in major reconstructions [1]. The high vascularity of the soft tissues in the oral cavity has allowed the use of free bone graft in the repair of oral cavity defects; but larger grafts increase the risk of bone resorption or failure of graft take. Hyperbaric oxygen therapy is currently being used to optimize bone healing. This procedure increases bone cellular activity and capillary ingrowth, inducing new bone formation and accelerating bone healing. The aim of this chapter is to present our experience with a series of patients with extensive mandibular defects where the use of autogenous free bone grafts along with hyperbaric oxygen therapy as an important adjuvant was beneficial to the outcome.This chapter also presents other alternatives for mandibular reconstruction.

2. Defect evaluation

In mandibular reconstruction, the restoration of bone continuity is not the only criteria for success. The ultimate goals constituting success is attaining near normal morphology and appropriate relation to the opposing jaw, adequate bone height and width, good facial contour and support for overlying soft tissue structures and restoration of jaw of function.

Bony reconstruction planning begins with evaluation of the patient's anatomy in order to define the full extent of the existing defect (both bone and soft tissues) and select the best reconstruction technique for each particular case. The size of the defect will define the magnitude of the reconstruction [2,3]. Some defects may not need to be restored to original size and shape. Loss of a significant portion of a mandibular ramus, for example, may be adequately managed by providing continuity from the condyle to the body of the mandible without restoring the coronoid process.

The quantity and quality of the soft tissues are both important when choosing the reconstructive method. The complete closure of the soft tissue without tension is essential for success. If the tissue is inadequate in quantity, the use of horizontal incisions in the periosteum must be used to guarantee tissue flexibility when needed. This ensures good (tension-free) repair, minimizes postoperative discomfort and reduces dehiscence (one of the most commonly observed complications after grafting in the oral cavity).

On the other hand, if the quantity of soft tissue is adequate but the quality is poor, the reconstruction will be compromised or limited. Tissue with extensive scarring provides a poor host bed for any grafting procedure. When considering the use of non-vascularized bone grafts, the ideal soft and hard tissue bed should have enough bulk, vascularity, and cellularity in order to permit bone graft incorporation. In several cases, tissue loss, scar contracture, and previous irradiation will hamper secondary reconstruction. In this setting, the use of hyperbaric oxygenation should always be considered, because it promotes vascularization and angiogenesis.

Preoperative radiographic evaluation of patients undergoing reconstructive bone surgery aims to evaluate the nature and extent of the lesion and provide the surgeon with anatomic mapping of important structures. Also, follow-up examinations to confirm healing and to discover complications at an early stage are paramount. The selection of the most appropriate imaging method in each case must take into account the diagnostic capability and cost-effectiveness. Radiographic analysis, computed tomography with three-dimensional (3D) images and magnetic resonance can provide important information. With the development of rapid prototyping methods, such as stereolithography, fused deposition modeling and selective laser sintering, 3D reconstruction based on biomodels have become indispensible tools both for mandibular resection and bony reconstruction.

The use of 3D biomodels, may help delineate the osteotomy area, improving the accuracy of marginal resection. Pre-modeling of reconstruction plates according to the mandibular anatomy is also facilitated. At the time of the secondary reconstruction, the individual plate gives the surgeon a clear direction where the bone should be ideally placed. Another important possibility with these models is the reproduction of the anatomy of the resected area based on mirror imaging of the contralateral side of the mandible. This procedure guides the surgeon as to where to cut the bone graft in the donor area and enhance visualization of the points to be remodeled in the graft prior to fixation to reproduce the new mandible.

3. Reconstruction plates

Mandibular reconstruction plates and screws (2.4 System) are the most widely used devices for mandibular reconstruction; however 2.0 plates can be used in selected cases. With the conventional fixation technique, the tightening of the screws presses the plate against the bone (load sharing). This pressure generates friction, which may contribute to resorption of the grafted bone. However, with the locking systems (load bearing), additional threads within the screw head allows the plate to be anchored to the intraosseous screw instead of being compressed onto the bone. This reduces interference to the bone blood supply underlying the plate, prevents bone pressure necrosis and decreases the potential for plate failure at the screw-bone interface. These plates and screws provide an excellent rigid frame construction with high mechanical stability which is extremely useful in bone grafting (Figures 1-6).

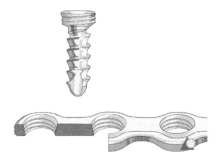

Figure 1. The locking plate has a corresponding threaded plate hole. Copyright by AO Foundation, Switzerland. Source: AO Surgery Reference, www.aosurgery.org.

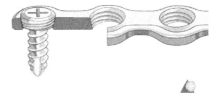

Figure 2. During insertion the locking head screw engages and locks into the threaded plate hole. Copyright by AO Foundation, Switzerland. Source: AO Surgery Reference, www.aosurgery.org.

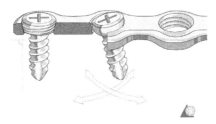

Figure 3. If necessary the threaded plate hole also accepts nonlocking screws, which permit greater angulation. Copyright by AO Foundation, Switzerland. Source: AO Surgery Reference, www.aosurgery.org.

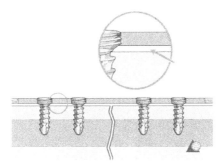

Figure 4. With the locking head screws engaged in the plate, the plate is not pressed onto the bone. This reduces interference to the blood supply to the bone underlying the plate. Copyright by AO Foundation, Switzerland. Source: AO Surgery Reference, www.aosurgery.org.

Reconstruction plates are usually shaped before the mandibular resection and applied afterwards. By bending these plates and placing drill holes in the proximal and distal mandible segments before complete mandibular resection, the surgeon can more confidently maintain the proper occlusion and relationships of the remaining mandibular segments after removal of the involved bone. Even in edentulous cases, this planning maintains a more natural contour and good joint function. With the currently available low-profile locking reconstruction plates, the contoured plate can closely approximate the natural mandibular projection without sacrificing durability and strength, even when used in conjunction with bone grafts. If, however, there is involvement of the buccal cortex of the mandible, direct plate contouring to the bone is not always possible. In these cases, removal of the buccal part of the lesion to allow plate positioning before complete resection is a possible option with satisfactory results. Post-resection freehand plate contouring and fixation is another possibility, however it is difficult, presumes the need of inter-maxillary fixation (IMF) and often yields suboptimal symmetry.

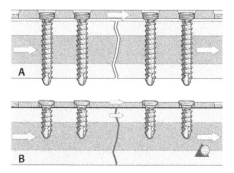

Figure 5. Loading forces are transmitted directly from the bone to the screws, then onto the plate, across the gap and again through the screws into the bone. Friction between plate and bone is not necessary for stability. The plate and screws provide adequate rigidity and do not depend on the underlying bone (load bearing osteosynthesis) when using a locking reconstruction plate 2.4. Copyright by AO Foundation, Switzerland. Source: AO Surgery Reference, www.aosurgery.org.

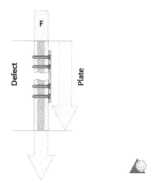

Figure 6. In load-bearing fixation the plate assumes 100% of the functional loads. Copyright by AO Foundation, Switzerland. Source: AO Surgery Reference, www.aosurgery.org.

It is important to understand the appropriate possibilities for bone graft fixation. In our experience, adequate internal fixation using reconstruction locking plates and, subsequently, free autogenous bone grafts seem to be most satisfactory.

4. Free bone grafting

During harvesting, tissue connections between the bone graft and surrounding tissues are transected. In the recipient site, the bone must be revitalized mainly via tissue ingrowth, although it is known that many cells within free bone grafts are able to survive after transplantation. The revitalization goes along with a process of initial remodeling and bone resorption, which is associated with bone volume loss. The amount of resorption depends on many factors, such as the quality of the bone (cortical, cancellous), bone graft fixation to surrounding bone, biomechanical properties (functional loading), the dimensions of the bone graft (it takes longer to revitalize large bone grafts, and therefore, usually they show greater percentage of bone loss) and tissue qualities at the recipient site (vascularization). The amount of bone formed is directly proportional to the number of viable osteogenic cells transferred. The next phase involves revascularization, remodeling, and reorganization of the previously formed bone by osteoblasts and osteoclasts.

Non-vascularized autogenous bone grafts can be harvested from the patient's calvarium, rib, ilium, tibia or fibula [4]. They can be successfully used for reconstruction of small to medium size mandibular defects with favorable prognosis. However, in large mandibular defects, bone reconstruction is still challenging.

Cancellous bone grafts, consisting of medullary bone and bone marrow, contain the highest percentage of viable cells. These grafts become rapidly vascularized due to their particulate structure and large surface area. In contrast, cortical grafts consisting of lamellar bone, provides more resistance to the graft. Cortico-cancellous bone grafts contain both cortical and underlying cancellous bone providing both viable cells and necessary strength for bridging discontinuous defects. The combination of particulate cortical bone and cancellous marrow provides the best potential for osteogenesis.

Bone harvesting should always be performed with sharp instruments under abundant irrigation, and the surgical time must be as short as possible to minimize tissue necrosis and preserve cell viability [5]. The same principles are required during the bone adaptation in the recipient site. The lack of adaptation of the bone block onto the recipient site and the presence of gaps can generate fibrous tissue interposition, which can be avoided with filling the gap with particulate autogenous bone, platelet rich plasma (PRP) or biomaterials.

The recipient site preparation should facilitate the subsequent adaptation of the graft and also expose the bone marrow, favoring revascularization, since the vessels from the periosteum were compromised when it was displaced. The cortical bone in the recipient site can be perforated or even removed with drills to enable contact of the marrow spaces of the graft [6].

Graft fixation is essential to allow its revascularization and incorporation. Movement of the bone block during the healing period results in fibrous tissue between the graft and the recipient site or graft resorption [5,6]. The fixation screws can be used in a passive or compressive manner, however, in the latter case, excessive compression must always be avoided. In cases of mandibular reconstruction decortication is extremely important before the placement of the grafts to support revascularization and facilitate the graft adaptation.

5. Hyperbaric oxygen therapy

The hyperbaric oxygen (HBO) is a therapeutic modality performed within devices called pressurized containers, in which the patient breathes pure oxygen at a high pressure. The HBO promotes an increase in the amount of dissolved oxygen in the blood due to increased pressure inside the chamber, aiding tissue oxygenation [7] (Figure 7).

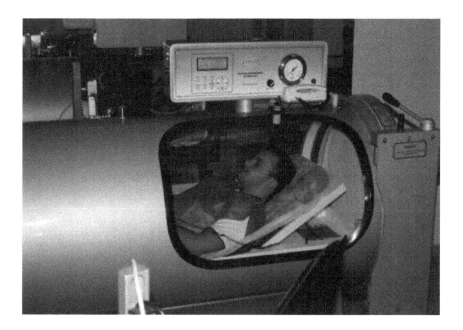

Figure 7. Patient in an HBO chamber during a hyperbaric oxygen therapy session.

For years, conventional medicine thought of HBO only as a treatment for decompression sickness and air embolism. However, the use of HBO is becoming increasingly common in general practice. HBO has already been used in the treatment of carbon monoxide poisoning, cerebral arterial gas syndrome, decompression sickness, osteoradionecrosis and clostridial gas gangrene. It is also beneficial to improve the healing of a variety of compromised or hypoxic wounds including diabetic ulcers, radiation-induced tissue damage, gangrene, and necrotizing anaerobic bacterial infections [8].

Complications of HBO can be due to either O_2 toxicity or barotrauma. O_2 toxicity is due to formation of superoxide, OH- and H_2O_2. Signs and symptoms of O_2 toxicity mainly involve respiratory system and central nervous system with symptoms like anxiety, nausea, vomiting, seizures, vertigo and decreased level of consciousness. Patients also show respiratory discomfort ranging from dry cough and substernal pain to pulmonary edema and fibrosis [7].

HBO is contraindicated in a patient with pneumothorax due to increased risk of gas embolism. It is also contraindicated in epileptics, hyperthermia and acidosis due to increased risk of seizures. Chronic obstructive pulmonary disease, malignant tumors, pregnancy, claustrophobia, hereditary spherocytosis and optic neuritis are other relative contraindications for the use of HBO therapy [9].

Following maxillofacial trauma there is a vascular disruption which leads to the formation of a hypoxic zone. While hypoxia is necessary to stimulate angiogenesis and revascularization, extended hypoxia will blunt the healing process. HBO may be used to aid in the healing of these compromised wounds by increasing oxygen diffusion from the capillaries to tissues [10]. The available oxygen also has bacteriostatic and bactericidal activites, enhances the phagocytic capacity of white blood cells and promotes differentiation of fibroblasts by interfering with the synthesis of collagen. Important biological events such as angiogenesis and osteogenesis are also stimulated by HBO [11], improving tissue repair and increasing the overall success of reconstruction procedures.

The stimulation of osteogenesis by HBO has been reported in animal experiments and clinical cases. In 1996, Sawai et al. conducted a study to evaluate the effect of hyperbaric oxygen therapy on autogenous free bone grafts transplanted from iliac crest to the mandibles of rabbits and the results indicate that HBO accelerates the union of autogenous free bone grafts [12]. Other studies also demonstrated that HBO elevates alkaline phosphatase activity, a marker of bone formation, in rats following mandibular osteotomy [13], increased osteoblastic activity and angiogenesis in irradiated mandibles undergoing distraction [14] and increased vascular endothelial growth factor expression during bone healing [15].

5.1. A hyperbaric oxygen protocol in mandibular reconstructions

The following treatment steps are included in these sessions: 10 minutes of ventilation to fill the chamber with 100% oxygen, 10 to 15 minutes of diving (0.06 to 0.12 kgf/cm² in 1 minute), the patients are exposed to 2.4 ATA (Atmosphere Absolute) pressure for 90 minutes, 10 minutes of re-surfacing and 10 minutes of air ventilation. HBO is given every day and the treatment starts 10 days before bony reconstruction and continues for another 40 days after the surgical procedure.

6. Clinical cases

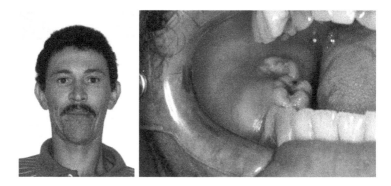

Figure 8. Patient with ossifying fibroma in the right side of the mandible. Extra and intra oral appearance.

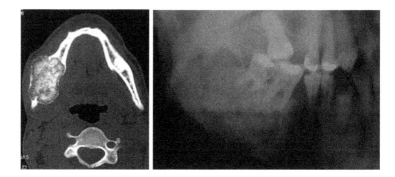

Figure 9. Computed Tomography and panoramic images revealing the lesion area.

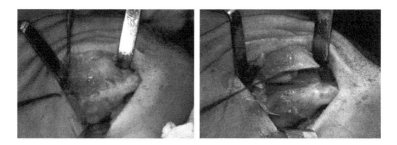

Figure 10. Part of the lesion was removed to permit reconstruction plate modeling maintaining mandibular contour.

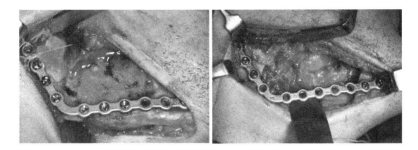

Figure 11. Reconstruction plate installation prior and after complete removal of the lesion. This preserves dental occlusion and condylar position.

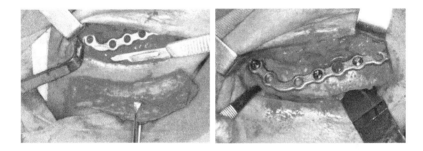

Figure 12. Mandibular reconstruction with free iliac bone 6 months after resection.

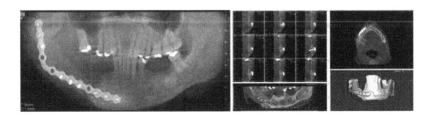

Figure 13. Computed Tomography images 8 months after bony reconstruction revealing the maintenance of bone graft volume. The next step is implant installation for final oral rehabilitation.

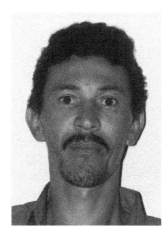

Figure 14. Extra-oral image 8 months after bony reconstruction showing preserved mandibular contour and facial symmetry.

6.1. Clinical case

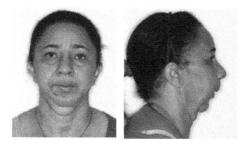

Figure 15. Patient sought treatment for mandibular reconstruction 5 years after undergoing surgery for removal of an ossifying fibroma. There was a significant impairment of the symmetry of the face and backward positioning of the soft tissues of the lower face ("Andy Gump" deformity).

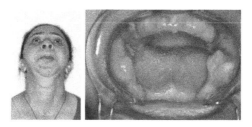

Figure 16. Intraoral image showing the soft tissue condition. There was difficulty in mouth opening.

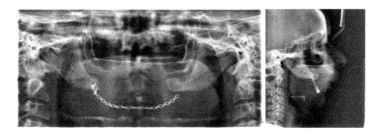

Figure 17. Radiographic images revealing failure of the fixation system and major deficiency in lower face position.

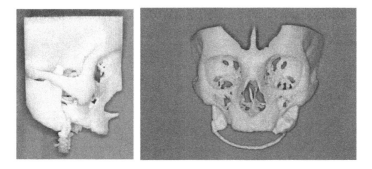

Figure 18. biomodels constructed to better understand the case and assist planning mandibular reconstruction.

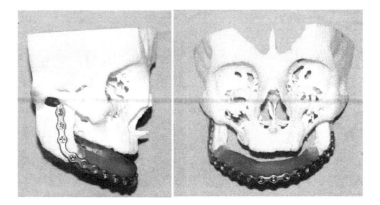

Figure 19. The 2.4 reconstruction plate was previously modeled to facilitate the surgery procedure and reduce operation time.

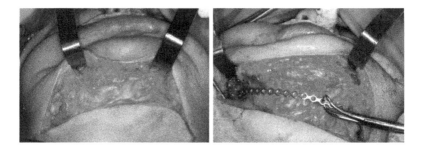

Figure 20. After the surgical approach, the 2.0 miniplate was removed and the bone segments located.

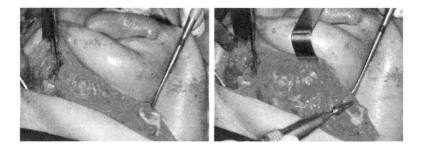

Figure 21. Refreshing the bone margins is important to enhance bone graft take.

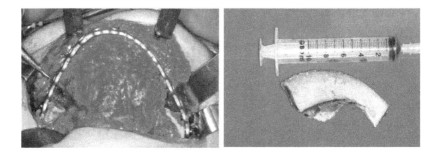

Figure 22. The locking plate was installed and the iliac crest bone was removed.

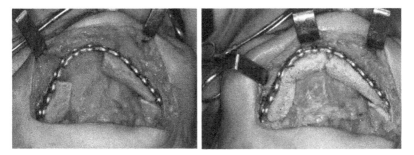

Figure 23. Positioned and fixed bone blocks. In this case the locking plate supports the full load.

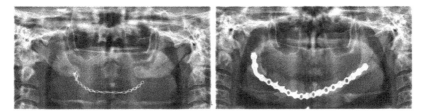

Figure 24. Pre and post-operative images of mandibular reconstruction.

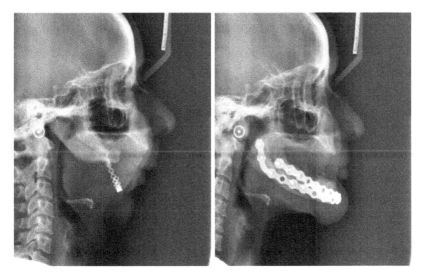

Figure 25. Pre and post-operative profile imagesof mandibular reconstruction.

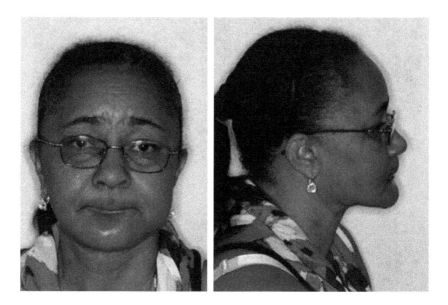

Figure 26. Postoperative appearance after mandibular reconstruction with preserved contour of the mandible and face.

7. Clinical case

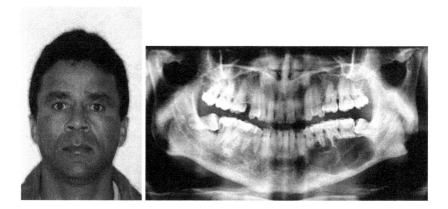

Figure 27. The patient was diagnosed with ameloblastoma in the left mandibular body. The panoramic radiograph shows an extensive multilocular lesion and resorption of tooth roots.

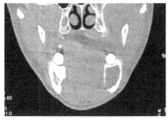
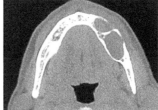

Figure 28. Computed Tomography images are important to define the extent of the affected area.

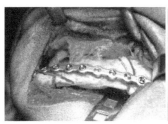
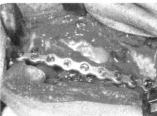

Figure 29. Installation of the 2.4 reconstruction plate before and after complete remove the lesion. These preserves dental occlusion and condylar position.

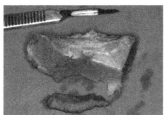
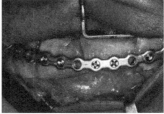

Figure 30. Mandibular reconstruction with iliac free bone 9 months after the resection.

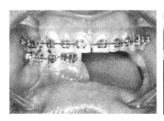
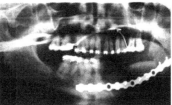

Figure 31. Intraoral examination evidenced good quality of soft tissue.Orthodontic brackets are installed to prevent extrusion of the upper teeth.Panoramic image 6 months after mandibular bony reconstruction demonstrating bone volume maintenance.

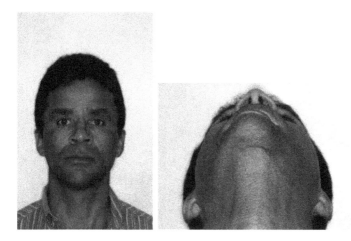

Figure 32. Postoperative appearance after mandibular reconstruction with preserved contour of the mandible and face.

7.1. Clinical case

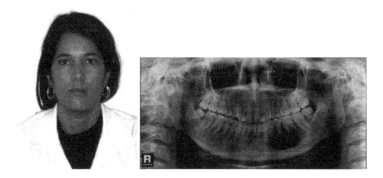

Figure 33. The patient was diagnosed with ameloblastoma in left mandibular body. The panoramic radiograph shows an extensive multilocular lesion and resorption of tooth roots.

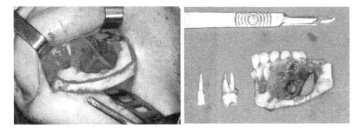

Figure 34. Marginal mandibular resection preserving the mandible basis.

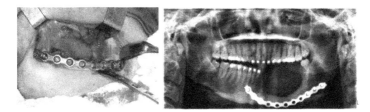

Figure 35. Installation of the 2.4 locking reconstruction plate. The presence of plate protects the jaw of a possible fracture.

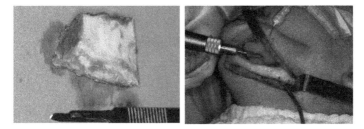

Figure 36. Mandibular bony reconstruction 8 months after resection. The receptor site of the graft should be prepared by removing part of the bone cortex. This favors the incorporation of the graft.

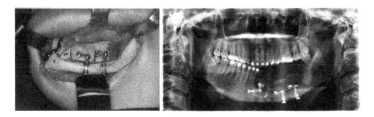

Figure 37. In this case, the reconstruction plate was removed and the bone blocks were fixed using 2.0 miniplates. The use of miniplates provided a better fit and positioning of the blocks.

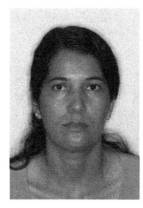
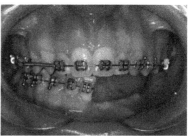

Figure 38. Postoperative appearance after mandibular reconstruction with preserved contour of the mandible and face. Intraoral examination evidenced good quality of soft tissue. Orthodontic brackets are installed to prevent extrusion of the upper teeth.

Author details

Maiolino Thomaz Fonseca Oliveira[1], Flaviana Soares Rocha[1], Jonas Dantas Batista[1], Sylvio Luiz Costa de Moraes[2] and Darceny Zanetta-Barbosa[1]

1 Department of Oral and Maxillofacial Surgery and Implantology – School of Dentistry - Federal University of Uberlândia – UFU, Brazil

2 Head, Clinic for Cranio-Maxillofacial Surgery at Hospital São Francisco. Director of Facial Reconstruction Center – RECONFACE. Faculty AO-Foundation

References

[1] Pogrel MA, Podlesh S, Anthony JP, Alexander J. A comparison of vascularised and nonvascularized bone grafts for reconstruction of mandibular continuity defects. J Oral Maxillofac Surg. 1997 Nov;55(11):1200-6.

[2] Bernstein S, Cooke J, Fotek P, Wang HL. Vertical bone augmentation: where are we now? Implant Dent. 2006 Sep;15(3):219-28. Review.

[3] McAllister BS, Haghighat K. Bone augmentation techniques. J Periodontol. 2007 Mar; 78(3):377-96.

[4] Weibull L, Widmark G, Ivanoff CJ, Borg E, Rasmusson L. Morbidity after chin bone harvesting--a retrospective long-term follow-up study. Clin Implant Dent Relat Res. 2009 Jun;11(2):149-57. Epub 2008 Jul 24.

[5] Cypher TJ, Grossman JP. Biological principles of bone graft healing. J Foot Ankle Surg. 1996 Sep-Oct;35(5):413-7.

[6] Buser D, Dula K, Hirt HP, Schenk RK. Lateral ridge augmentation using autografts and barrier membranes: a clinical study with 40 partially edentulous patients. J Oral Maxillofac Surg. 1996 Apr;54(4):420-32; discussion 432-3.

[7] Brazilian Society of Hyperbaric Medicine (SBMH), 2010.

[8] DESOLA J, CRESPO A, GARCIA A et al: Indicaciones y Contraindicaciones de la Oxigenoterapia Hiperbarica. Nº 1260, 5- 11 de Junho de JANO/Medicina, 1998;LIV.

[9] Fernandes TD. [Hyperbaric medicine]. Acta Med Port. 2009 Jul-Aug;22(4):323-34. Epub 2009 Aug 10. Review. Portuguese.

[10] Feldmeier JJ. Hyperbaric oxygen for delayed radiation injuries. Undersea Hyperb Med. 2004 Spring; 31(1):133-45.

[11] Jacobson AS, Buchbinder D, Hu K, Urken ML. Paradigm shifts in the management of osteoradionecrosis of the mandible. Oral Oncol. 2010 Nov;46(11):795-801. Epub 2010 Sep 16. Review.

[12] Sawai T, Niimi A, Takahashi H, Ueda M. Histologic study of the effect of hyperbaric oxygen therapy on autogenous free bone grafts. J Oral Maxillofac Surg. 1996 Aug; 54(8):975-81.

[13] Nilsson LP. Effects of hyperbaric oxygen treatment on bone healing. An experimental study in the rat mandible and the rabbit tibia. Swed Dent J 1989;64(1):1-33.

[14] Muhonen A, Haaparanta M, Gronroos T, Bergman J, Knuuti J, Hinkka S, et al. Osteoblastic activity and neoangiogenesis in distracted bone of irradiated rabbit mandible with or without hyperbaric oxygen treatment. Int J Oral Maxillofacial Surg 2004;33(2):173-8.

[15] Fok TC, Jan A, Peel SA, Evans AW, Clokie CM, Sándor GK. Hyperbaric oxygen results in increased vascular endothelial growth factor (VEGF) protein expression in rabbit calvarial critical-sized defects. Oral Surg Oral Med Oral Pathol Oral Radiol Endod. 2008 Apr;105(4):417-22.

Chapter 6

Maxillofacial Reconstruction of Ballistic Injuries

Mohammad Hosein Kalantar Motamedi,
Seyed Hossein Mortazavi, Hossein Behnia,
Masoud Yaghmaei, Abbas Khodayari,
Fahimeh Akhlaghi, Mohammad Ghasem Shams and
Rashid Zargar Marandi

Additional information is available at the end of the chapter

1. Introduction

This chapter presents our experience with treatment of facial fractures and defects subsequent to various ballistic injuries based on experience gained from management of numerous warfare injuries during the Iraq-Iran war and thereafter (1986-2013).

2. Presentation

The clinical presentation and devastation of penetrating injuries of the face resulting from ballistic weaponry varies according to the caliber of the weapon used, the distance from which the victim is shot and velocity of the projectile. Projectiles from ballistic weaponry may be either high-velocity or low- velocity.

2.1. High-velocity projectiles

High-velocity projectiles to the face have devastating functional and esthetic consequences because they shatter and scatter the bones and teeth. The entry wound is usually small while the exit wound is large and management is difficult.

2.2. Low-velocity projectiles

Low-velocity projectiles are usually less devastating with regard to fracture pattern and tissue damage ; therefore management of these injuries is usually less complicated.

3. Management

Generally, treatment of ballistic injuries mandate prompt assessment and early comprehensive management in the first operation [1-3]. However, some [4,5] feel that delayed reconstruction of ballistic injuries, avoidance of mini-plates, use of small incisions, minimal exposure of bony fragments, external pin fixations, and avoidance of intraosseous wiring is safer (fearing necrosis, infection and other complications).

3.1. Controversies in comprehensive management: Early vs. delayed intervention

3.1.1. Proponents of delayed intervention

Ballistic wounds are considered contaminated and this is why some are against early intervention and comprehensive management at the first operation. Advocates of delayed intervention state that delayed repair ensures a clean, segregated wound bed [5].

3.1.2. Proponents of early intervention

Those in favor of early intervention and comprehensive management at the first operation state that delay causes problems such as contracture scars, deformity, displacement of bone segments (due to muscle pull), difficulty in fracture reduction, patient anxiety, longer hospital stay and an additional operation to reopen the same wound (closed hastily at the field hospital, nearest emergency post or local hospital before transfer) in order to graft the hard or soft tissues [6,7].

In the maxillofacial region many ballistic injuries may be treated early; and several authors have opposed the strategy of universally delaying all surgical interventions of facial ballistic injuries suggesting a more comprehensive surgical operation can be done primarily in many [2,6 8]. Good results following acute treatment of projectile facial wounds during a 4-year period in the Afghan war has been reported more recently. Definitive and comprehensive treatment of ballistic facial injuries in the first stage with minimal debridement has been shown to result in better restoration of the facial deformity, lower morbidity, faster return of function, shorter hospital stay, and one less operation for the patient (when bone continuity was obtained)[2,7,9,10]. Additional advantages of early single-stage repair include a fresh wound, ability to expose and locate displaced fracture segments upon debridement, easier anatomic reduction of facial fractures (no fibrosis), facilitated arch bar placement, facilitated fracture manipulation reduction and osteosynthesis (no contractures) and definitive soft-tissue management. Moreover, it also allows for restoration of occlusion, salvaging loose teeth, a more expedient return of function and closer restoration of pre-injury appearance postoperatively [9,10].

3.2. Injury assessment

Ballistic injuries to the face must be assessed and addressed with regard to the wounds sustained, the injury profile and general status of the patient to decide when and how to treat. The criteria which dictate when to operate are discussed in this chapter as are the results, outcomes, and benefits of treating both hard and soft tissues in the first operation (early comprehensive management).

4. Early comprehensive management of ballistic injuries to the face

From 1991 to 2012 we treated 51 patients aged 8 – 50 years (mean 24.4±7.8 yrs.) for ballistic injuries of the face; 30 were rendered early comprehensive management based on indication.

4.1. Indications for early intervention to treat both hard and soft tissue ballistic injuries at the first operation

Early intervention and comprehensive management was done when there was:

- No gross infection

- No bone comminution to preclude osteosynthesis

- No extensive soft tissue loss to preclude bone coverage

- No general health problems such as medical instability or moribund patient

- No need for major grafting

- No concomitant more serious or life-threatening injuries requiring urgent attention

In these cases, acute management aimed to treat both hard and soft tissue injuries definitively at the first operation to restore arch continuity; because occlusion, form, function and esthetics can be restored later provided that continuity has been restored.

4.2. Contraindications for early intervention to treat both hard and soft tissue ballistic injuries in the first operation

Early intervention and comprehensive management was not done when there was:

- Gross infection

- Concomitant more serious injury or multiple injuries of higher priority

- Poor general health

- Pulverized bone precluding fixation

- Extensive loss of soft-tissue (requiring distant flaps)
- Requirment for large bone grafts

4.3. Treatment procedure (inside-out and bottom-up)

Thirty patients with maxillofacial ballistic injuries underwent early intervention to treat both hard and soft tissues at the first operation; basic treatment included:

a. General anesthesia, nasoendotracheal intubation and throat pack placement

b. Extensive oral and extraoral irrigation (dilute hydrogen peroxide + povidone iodide followed by normal saline), brushing the teeth and debridement of facial wounds.

c. Arch bar placement (in dentate patients), establishing occlusion and temporary maxillo-mandibular fixation (MMF)

d. Removal of floating fragments (teeth particles, debris, and shell fragments) while salvaging bone; tooth roots within the alveolus were not extracted at this stage nor were mobile teeth.

e. Locating the scattered bone segments within the wound and using them to restore bone continuity especially in the mandible.

f. Removal of temporary MMF and removal of throat pack.

g. Placement of MMF.

h. Wound closure in layers following irrigation (from the inside-out) using 3-0 polygalactin, 4-0 polygalactin and 5-0 nylon sutures respectively.

Note: In addition to arch bars, titanium miniplates or wires were used as necessary following fracture reduction.

- In all dentate cases, arch bars were first placed and intermaxillary fixation (temporary MMF) was done prior to bone reduction to re-establish the occlusion. Then, the fractured and scattered bone segments were realigned and fixated using miniplates, lag screws, reconstruction plates, or titanium trays (Figure 1 A-D). Final MMF was placed after removal of the throat pack.
- Arch bar placement with MMF but without osteosynthesis was possible when the reduced bone segments contained teeth.
- High velocity ballistic wounds cause fracture and dispersion of teeth, bone, foreign bodies and debris into the lips, tongue, cheeks, and elsewhere; these sites were visualized, palpated and searched prior to wound closure.
- Projectiles beyond the depth of the wound and not within reach were not sought.
- After management of the hard tissues, soft tissue injuries were treated by debridement and primary wound closure performed loosely in layers from the inside out, using common local flap techniques to compensate for the tissue loss.

• In cases with bone comminution the soft tissues were closed and bone graft was done 3 – 4 weeks later when wounds had healed.

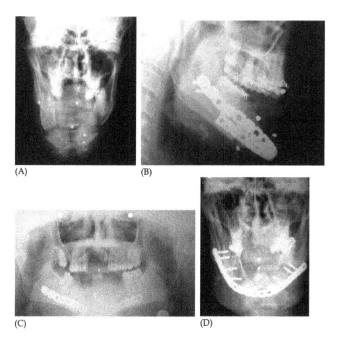

(A)   (B)

(C)   (D)

Figure 1. (A) Posterior–anterior skull radiograph of a typical patient shot in the face revealing multiple fragments of the mandible displaced inferiorly into the neck due to suprahyoid muscle pull. First arch bars and MMF and then a reconstruction plate were placed. (B) Lateral view after location, reduction of segments, and screw fixation of bone fragments ; large bone segments were secured to the reconstruction plate restoring continuity and chin projection. Smaller segments were wedged in place. (C) Panoramic view 6 months later showing bone consolidation and restoration of bone continuity. Had this not been done another operation to bone graft the mandible would have been necessary again with MMF. (D). PA view postoperatively. Note bone segments, reduced and fixed by 2.7mm screws in order to obtain mandibular continuity.

5. Clinical course

Thirty of 51 patients were treated for both hard and soft tissues injuries at the first operation (comprehensive intervention). Patient ages ranged from 8 to 50 years (mean 24.4±7.8 years). All patients were male. The mandible was injured in 96% and the maxilla in 54%; 22% required tracheotomy; 91% had isolated facial injuries with no other body area injured; 64% were managed in a single definitive early operation and 36% required two major operations. In the acute group, 6/30 patients had minor complications such as scarring and wound discharge. Transient postoperative discharge from the flap suture site was noted in these patients; this resolved within several weeks following daily irrigation and cleansing of the wound site. The procedures in these patients are shown in Table 1.

Early comprehensive intervention for firearm injuries to the face was effective in all 30 selected cases. This resulted in restoration of occlusion and continuity of the jaw, fixation of luxated or extruded teeth, early return of function, prevention of segment displacement due to tissue contracture, less scarring, and no need for major bone graft reconstruction later on [Table 2]. Flap healing was favorable in all patients. None of the patients had major complications (i.e., necrosis or osteomyelitis).

Procedure and type of fracture fixation	Percentage
Primary debridement + open fracture reduction (without wire, plate, or screw osteosynthesis) + wound closure	62.5 %
Primary debridement + open reduction (with wire, plate, or screw osteosynthesis) + wound closure	37.5 %

Table 1. Type of fracture fixation used in 30 patients treated via early comprehensive intervention in the first operation.

Those not treated primarily were only debrided and had arch bars placed. Definitive treatment of hard and soft tissue management was rendered in another subsequent operation after soft tissues and defects had healed. At that time, bone reduction was difficult because of scarring, and displacement of remaining segments (due to muscle pull especially in the chin, mandibular angle and ramus where medial displacement was common). Reduction of extruded and displaced teeth was also difficult and often not feasible. Wound edges were inverted and required undermining. No significant differences however, were noted in terms of infection or other major complications following early or delayed intervention [Table 2].

Treatment	Displaced / extruded or intruded teeth	Healing	Fracture reduction and fixation	Wound Bed	Contracture	Hospital stay	Arch bar placement and occlusion	Anxiety	Ability to expose / locate
Early	Can be placed back into the socket and into occlusion	Primary	Easy	Fresh	Not seen	Shorter	Easier	Less	Easier
Delayed	Often cannot be placed in the socket or into occlusion	Secondary	Difficult	Often granulated requiring refreshing of tissue borders	Seen often	Longer	More difficult	Greater	More difficult

Table 2. Comparison of benefits of early comprehensive intervention versus delayed intervention in management of maxillofacial ballistic injuries.

In some injuries primary treatment may not be indicated nor possible (ie.brain edema) see Figure 2.

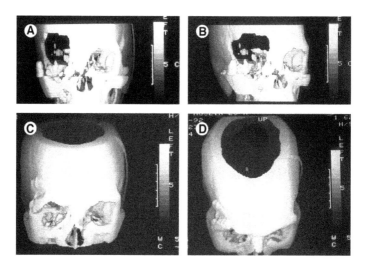

Figure 2. (A) Three-dimensional computed tomography scan of an extensive high-velocity bullet wound exiting the right orbit and anterior skull. (B) Note the amount of damage that may be inflicted by high-velocity projectiles. (C and D) After neurosurgery, reconstruction of the hard tissues was done via iliac bone grafts.

6. Discussion

There is no consensus on the timing of treatment for bone and soft tissue injuries resulting from firearms. The conventional method is primary closure, serial debridements and definitive reconstruction at a later stage. An alternative to this approach is immediate definitive surgical intervention and reconstruction at the first operation [11-17]. The presence of concomitant injuries of the body, fear of postoperative infection, unavailability of surgical hardware and lack of surgical experience in the treatment of penetrating ballistic injuries are among the factors that had created supporters for delayed treatment [2]. The use of external fixators have been recommended by some [4]; but in our unit we find them to be bulky and uncomfortable. They also add additional scars to the already damaged face. Our study shows that ballistic jaw fractures can often be reduced, immobilized, and fixed in occlusion at the time of the first operation along with primary closure and internal fixation with less trauma (provided that soft tissue coverage is feasible and MMF is used). If reconstruction plates are used MMF may be omitted [16,18].

6.1. Rationale for primary comprehensive management of hard and soft tissues at the time of the first operation

In our unit, we aim to restore bone continuity primarily (especially in the mandible). Because, if integrity of the jaw is restored, subsequent operations are facilitated for both the patient and surgeon and because MMF will not be needed again in subsequent operations. Additionally, when intervention is delayed, a myriad of problems set in:

- Fibrosis occurs around bone segments and makes locating and mobilizing them difficult or predisposes them to necrosis.

- Bone edges round-off (we cannot fix the puzzle) and will require refreshening upon reconstruction (for bone graft take).

- Restoration of pre-injury form and function in jaws without continuity is more difficult in delayed patients as the remaining segments often become displaced due to muscle pull (i.e., medial and superior rotational displacement of the mandibular ramus and posterior-inferior displacement of the chin). This makes reduction extremely difficult due to fibrosis and contracture.

- Release of this fibrotic tissue is necessary to reduce fracture segments; this requires stripping the tissues off the bone segments thus devitalizing them.

Often in high velocity facial injuries, the hard tissues are found to be scattered and displaced rather than avulsed. Locating and securing them in place is better than aggressive debridement to remove them in fear of sequestration and infection. Because, doing so, devitalizes and strips the fragments from their vital attachments. Often tracking the path of the projectile to the fracture facilitates finding segments of fractured bone. The bone segments can then be manipulated and wedged into their proper place after locating them at the very time of wound debridement. The bone although fragmented is fresh at that time and more likely to take. Upon primary intervention, projectiles not within reach via the wound bed are disregarded as exploration for these foreign bodies is often unnecessary and may be detrimental for the patient [2,16]. Arch bars, titanium miniplates or wire osteosynthesis were applied when necessary following open reduction along with MMF [Table 1]. All fractures do not require internal fixation however. Arch bar placement and restoration of occlusion following open reduction followed by MMF is sometimes adequate [2]. This is often possible when fractured bone segments contain teeth. Sali Bukhari recently reported on facial gunshot wounds. He found facial gunshot wounds to frequently involve the mandible and reiterated that early management of gunshot wounds not only results in better esthetics, reduced hospital stay and early return to function, but also to a better psychosocial profile preventing depression; when the patient has to tolerate the mutilated face and defective jaw for several days or longer until definitive treatment is rendered he no doubt suffers. The latter is an important issue of concern often overlooked and not addressed in most studies [18].

6.2. Overview of consequences inherent to delayed management

Inherent consequences of delayed management inlude:

- Loss of loose or extruded teeth (which cannot be placed back into the alveolus after delay of several days or more and may not take).

- Problems in restoring occlusion

- Difficulty in fracture reduction due to callus formation

- Displacement of bone segments due to contracture and muscle pull

- Excessive granulation tissue formation and fibrosis of wounds

- Problems in eating due to untreated wound

- Anxiety due to deformity, anticipation of treatment and uncertainty

- Scarring and less esthetic outcome

- Increased cost and length of hospital stay

- An additional major operation

6.3. Hard tissue management

Vayvada *et al.* treated 15 patients with high-energy bullet wounds. The conventional approach with delayed reconstruction was done for 10 patients and immediate definitive surgical reconstruction for 5 patients. They stated that immediate reconstruction eliminated the disadvantages of the conventional method such as high infection rate, high scarring rate and deformities resulting from contraction of tissues (similar to our findings)[13]. In our series, 22% of our patients required tracheotomies. This compared well with that found by Hollier *et al.*, where 21% of all facial fractures required a tracheostomy [9]. In all cases, in our series arch bars were placed with MMF prior to bone reduction to ensure proper occlusion. MMF postoperatively prevents chronic osteomyelitis or nonunion *via* preventing movement of segments. The application of arch bars for gunshot injuries of the jaws is the mainstay of treatment to re-establish arch form, occlusion and dentoalveolar stability.

6.4. Soft tissue management

Local undermining and the use of regional soft-tissue advancement rotation flaps for primary closure of maxillofacial soft tissue defects during the first operation has proved beneficial from both an esthetic and functional point of view [2,11,13,19]. Leaving defects open results in extensive scarring of the facial tissues and complicates subsequent surgical procedures, and should be avoided even in contaminated penetrating wounds [2,11,13,16,19]. In such situations, debridement and loose closure of the tissues transferred locally followed by administration of antibiotics may be a better alternative [2,11,13,14].

6.5. Antibiotics

Antibiotic therapy plays a major role in the prevention of infection of both hard and soft-tissues; early and appropriate surgical debridement, copious irrigation, fixation and immobilization of injured tissues, detailed wound closure, drainage, maintenance of clean dressings, nutrition, tetanus prophylaxis, and restoration of circulating fluid volume are equally important in ballistic injuries [2,11,13,16,19]. Soft tissue healing is usually favorable in patients with penetrating facial injuries; however, postoperative discharge from the suture sites may be seen.

This usually resolves within several weeks after daily irrigation with dilute povidone iodine or hydrogen peroxide solutions. Form and function of the soft tissue reconstructed regions recover usually within a year postoperatively. The esthetic results that can be obtained are generally acceptable to patients [2,11,13,14].

6.6. General health

The general health status of the wounded patient is important. The hemodynamic of the patient must be addressed early on as the oxygen carrying capacity is influential in both wound healing and prevention of infection in injured victims who have suffered extensive blood loss. This issue may warrant delayed intervention especially in the light of more serious concomitant injuries [2,7,11,14].

6.7. Mental health

The emotional conditions of patients with facial ballistic injuries have been evaluated and major depression signs have been reported. Functional evaluation has shown a significant correlation between facial appearance after reconstruction and social activity level [16-18]. Thus, the sooner the surgical treatment is rendered the sooner the psychological recovery.

6.8. Revisions

Revisions and secondary operations are often necessary and were performed in 36% of our patients following the first operation. Revisions are usually needed to remove scars, etc. near the eyes, the alar base of the nose, oral commissures and the vermilion border of the lips. Many of these and other operations including masticatory rehabilitation and restoration of occlusion with osseointegrated implants can be done later under local anesthesia and sedation on an out-patient basis [14,16,20].

7. Summary

The resultant injury from ballistic wounds are diverse because of the variability of the projectile, its motion, velocity, and the characteristics of the tissues involved. When a high-velocity projectile strikes the jaw, often the wound will consist of a severely comminuted mandible surrounded by damaged soft tissues and implanted multiple foreign bodies. This presents a challenge for the treating surgeon. The anatomy and function of the jaw is such that the care of the gunshot wound requires a combination of trauma surgery and reconstructive surgeries. There are varying techniques advocated for the management of ballistic wounds to the face. However, for the comminuted fracture sustained from a ballistic wound, an approach involving intermaxillary fixation, wound debridement and immediate management using a comprehensive approach that can restore function and esthetics. This approach to the comminuted jaw has led to the effective management provided communition is not extensive. The complication rate is comparable with the current literature and provides many advantages mainly a 1-stage major operation to restore appropriate function and cosmesis to the patient. [12,14,16].

7.1. Surgical Intervention in ballistic injuries

Ballistic wounds are associated with a high incidence of maxillofacial injuries requiring surgical intervention. Many may be treated acutely and definitively with procedures designed to repair both the hard and soft tissue injuries simultaneously to restore bony continuity (especially in the mandible), restoration of esthetics and function using the tissues within or adjacent to the wound. This is advocated because if continuity of the mandible can be obtained subsequent operations will not need maxillomandibular fixation again. Additionally, the course of healing is not disrupted with another subsequent operation (in the same wound) and because it may decrease hospital stay without increasing patient morbidity in patients selected for this intervention. Moreover, residual defects can be treated later as out-patient procedures.

7.1.1. Soft-tissue reconstruction

Soft-tissue reconstruction of facial defects and deformities following ballistic injury is not always an easy or straightforward procedure. The limited availability of adjacent skin, the complex function, contours, texture and intricate innervation of the face, especially in the area of the eyes and the lips, along with the many facial esthetic subunits make the goals of restoring function and esthetics challenging and often difficult to achieve [21]. Local flaps utilize tissue that abuts the defect requiring coverage. These flaps are used to cover skin defects in areas without enough tissue laxity to afford primary closure. The donor site for a local flap ideally should have enough laxity to allow primary repair in addition to providing tissue to the recipient site for coverage of the defect.

In victims of ballistic injuries, the difficulty in application of standard soft-tissue transfer techniques to treat facial defects, is compounded by devastation resulting from high-velocity projectiles in a patient with often multiple, concomitant injuries. Thus, reconstruction is more problematic because of extensive tissue mutilation, edema, compromised blood supply and the involvement of the underlying hard-tissues compounded by the contaminated nature of ballistic wounds [19,22]. Despite these facts, attempting simple closure may often prove adequate to treat the resultant defect or deformity (Figure 3).

However, in complicated cases with extensive tissue loss we face more dilemmas [2,19]. Appreciation of basic flap techniques, as well as applicable modifications and combinations of different flaps can prove invaluable to the maxillofacial surgeon confronted by ballistic injuries, allowing for a more acceptable cosmetic and functional result. In this section we present the application of several useful local flap combinations used to reconstruct various-sized, full-thickness facial defects and deformities in patients with ballistic injuries and discuss applications of local flaps in several facial subunits.

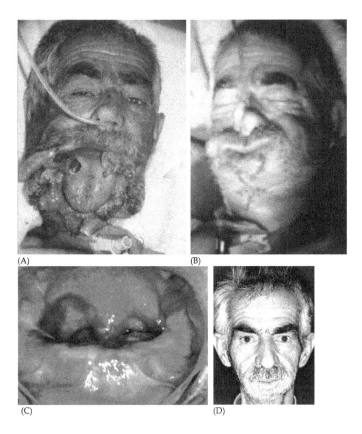

Figure 3. (A) View of the patient on admission, depicting extensive hard and soft tissue destruction by the exiting projectile (B) Immediate postoperative photograph. (C) Twelve months after bone grafting the mandible with iliac bone chips in titanium mesh and ridge augmentation. (D)Facial form and function has been restored.

7.1.2. Soft-tissue procedures

The soft-tissue procedures used were basically local-advancement or rotation-advancement flaps, used in conjunction with pedicled fat or subcutaneous supporting flaps, nasolabial, cheek, cervical, Dieffenbach and Abbe-type flaps. Scar revision, tissue repositioning, and lengthening procedures, such as W, V-Y, Z, or multiple Z-plasty techniques were used both primarily and secondarily depending on the individual case.

Thirty-three patients suffering ballistic injuries were treated at our department from 1986 to 2012. There were 32 males and 1 female patient, aged between 8 and 53 years, with an average age of 24.18 years. Bullets were the most common cause(70%), followed by shrapnel (21%), land mines (6%), and one breech block injury (3%). All patients included in this study had full thickness soft-tissue defects and were seen 1-3 days after the initial injury. The soft-tissue injuries involved the anatomical facial subunits (orbital, infraorbital, buccal,zygomatic, labial, mental and parotidomasseteric). At the operation, after hard tissues were addressed the soft-tissue injuries were treated by debridement and primary closure by combining, modifying, and tailoring standard local flap techniques to fit the location of the injury and compensate for the tissue loss.

The operations were classified regionally: the perioral region was involved in 15 cases (45%), the midface and cheeks were involved in 13 cases (39%), and the periorbital area was involved in 5 cases (15%). Local advancement flaps were applied initially for the majority of the patients (48%) followed by Z-plasty (39%) listed in Table 3.

Soft Tissue Procedure	Number
Cutaneous local advancement flaps	18
Cervicofacial advancement flaps	4
Zygomaticofacial advancement flaps	2
Preauricular advancement flap	1
Columellar reconstruction	1
Tissue rearrangement	8
Mucosal finger flaps	2
Double Abbe flap	1
Commissuroplasty	5
Pedicled fat flap	1
Supporting flaps	5
Dieffenbach flap	1
Nasolabial flaps	4
Perialar flap	1
Skin graft	1
Abbe flap	1
Z-plasty	13
V-Y-plasty	3
W-plasty	1
Palatal flap	1
Direct lip repair	1
Strip graft	1

Table 3. List of basic soft-tissue procedures used to treat maxillofacial ballistic soft-tissue injuries. Cutaneous local advancement flaps followed by Z-plasty procedures were most commonly used.

7.1.2.1. Perioral reconstruction

Three basic factors were considered prior to perioral reconstruction: (1) utilization of the remaining portions of the injured lips if possible; (2) using the opposite lip as the next resort when there was inadequate tissue for repair; and (3) use of local flaps from the sides of the defect.

- When as much as one-quarter of the lip was missing, direct linear closure, Z-plasty, or double Z-plasty (to prevent notching of the vermilion) was done. Larger defects of the lips and perioral regions were treated using flaps.

- When reconstruction with flaps was contemplated, several options were considered depending on the lip involved and amount of tissue loss:

Lateral defects of the lips

For lateral defects of up to one-third of the upper or lower lip, treatment usually utilized nasolabial flaps, a lateral flap combined with vermilion advancement (Figure 4), or the Abbe Estlander flap.

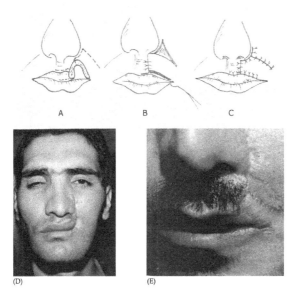

Figure 4. (A) Lateral defect of the upper lip with a nasolabial flap outlined for repair, (B) The nasolabial flap is transposed and the vermillion border of the upper lip is advanced laterally to the corner of the mouth, (C) Closure leaving inconspicuous scars in the philtrum, nasolabial, and alar fold. (D) A patient with a lateral upper lip defect resulting from a bullet. (E) View after treatment with a modified nasolabial flap and commisuroplasty. The maxillomandibular fractures were treated earlier.

We used a modified Abbe technique whenever possible, to preclude the need for a subsequent commisuroplasty (Figure 5).

Midline defects of the lips

For midline defects of the upper lip, treatment by direct advancement of the remaining portions of the lip with perialar excisions or an Abbe flap, taken from the midline of the lower lip and rotated 180 °, was used.

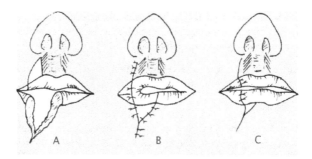

Figure 5. (A) Outline of the modified Abbe flap to repair a moderate-sized defect of the lower lip. (B) A triangular section of the upper lip is rotated to repair the lower lip defect. (C) The pedicle is sectioned two weeks later (note the commissures are spared).

Lower lip defects

Small-to-moderate sized defects of the lower lip were treated similarly. Lateral rotation or Abbe flaps, Z or V-Y plasties, were used (Figure 6).

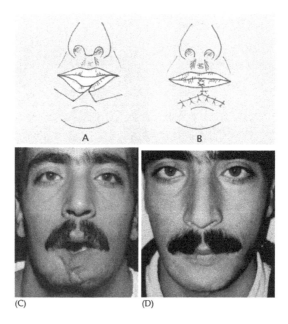

Figure 6. (A) Medial defect of the lower lip causing unsightly retraction. (B) Correction by lateral advancement flaps and V-Y plasty. (C) A patient with a gunshot wound defect of the chin, lower lip, and labiomental fold. (D) View of the patient after treatment of maxillomandibular fractures, iliac bone grafting, advancement flaps, V-Y, and Z-plasties.

In cases of complete loss of the lower lip and labiomental soft tissues, we combined bilateral Dieffenbach flaps with double Abbe flaps of the upper lip, and a cervical advancement flap, which proved relatively functional and effective in restoring lip competence and lip seal (Figure 7).

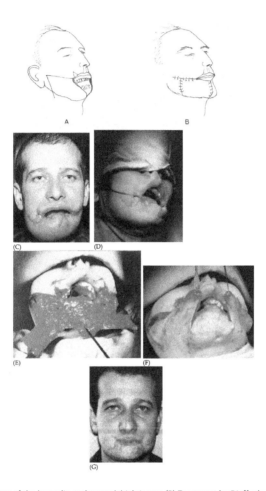

Figure 7. (A) Total defect of the lower lip and mentolabial tissues. (B) Treatment by Dieffenbach flaps, advancement of the full-thickness bilateral cheek flaps, and double Abbe flaps. (C) A similar defect in a gunshot patient with previously reconstructed hard tissues and soft tissue closure. The total loss of the lower lip and mentolabial tissues caused constant, intolerable, salivary drooling. The mandible was reconstructed primarily by fixing the fragmented bone segments to a reconstruction plate In the first operation,(same patient whose radiographs are shown in Figure 1). (D) Outline of the Dieffenbach flap used to reconstruct the lower lip. (E) Flap mobilization with double Abbe flaps outlined. (F) Flaps made passive for advancement. (G) 6-month postoperative photograph of the patient, showing restoration of lip competence.

Superficial deformities of the lips

Superficial deformities or residual defects which often occur with contraction of linear scars can distort the contour of the lip vermilion or cause notching. These were effectively treated by scar excision, re-creation of the defect, tissue rearrangement combined with supporting flaps, and Z- or V-Y plasty procedures, which proved useful when tissue lengthening was required (Figure 8).

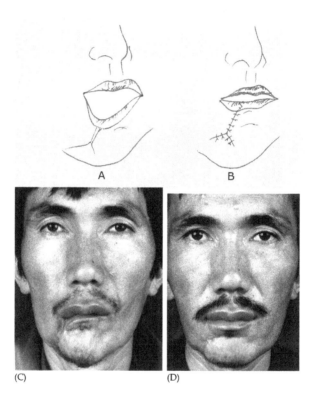

Figure 8. (A) Scarring and distortion of a lower lip defect. (B) Correction by scar excision, recreation of the defect, full-thickness lateral flap advancement, and V-Y and Z-plasty. (C) Gunshot patient with a similar contracture deformity. (D) After treatment. The right hemimandible was reconstructed using iliac bone marrow graft in a titanium mesh tray prior to this procedure.

7.1.2.2. Midface and cheek reconstruction

For reconstruction in cases with defects of the cheeks, zygomatic, and midfacial areas, the lateral cheek advancement or rotation flap was used. Transfer of tissue was based on the laxity found in the preauricular tissues, the lower face, and the neck. The larger the defect, the more

extensive the flap preparation. The deep surface of the flap was anchored to the soft tissue, and sometimes included the periosteum over the malar area, to help prevent traction on the eyelid (Figure 9).

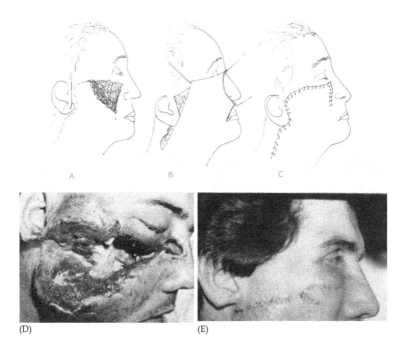

(D)   (E)

Figure 9. (A) Outline of a cervicofacial cheek flap for an avulsion defect. (B) Flap mobilization. (C) Reconstruction. (D) A patient with an extensive, deep avulsion defect of the right cheek and zygomatic area due to a high-velocity shrapnel. (E) View of the patient 1 week after the second surgical stage, note the previous scars of the cervicofacial-zygomatico-facial cheek advancement flap and primary closure in the preauricular area are still slightly visible.

This procedure was sometimes combined with a superiorly based nasolabial flap when ectropion was eminent. Smaller defects of the cheeks were treated with local undermining combined with Z-plastics and pedicled fat or subcutaneous supporting flaps to fill the defects and restore the natural prominence of the cheek.

7.1.2.3. Periorbital reconstruction

Reconstruction of defects of the lower eyelid or upper cheek basically employed the versatile nasolabial flap. For defects of this area, the pedicle of this flap was based superiorly, on the angular artery and rotated 90 ° to close the defect. The tip of the flap was anchored at the corner under the eyelid giving added support to the lower eyelid. This flap was also used to treat lower lid ectropion (Figure 10).

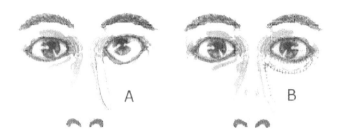

Figure 10. (A) Outline of a nasolabial flap for treatment of lower lid sagging and ectropion. (B) Reconstruction.

7.1.3. Hard-tissue injuries

Hard tissues were usually treated primarily along with closure of the soft-tissue injuries (76%). These procedures varied from debridement only (16%),primary debridement, closed reduction, and fixation (45%), primary debridement, open reduction and wire osteosynthesis (12%), or via primary debridement, open reduction and plate osteosynthesis (3%). When soft-tissue loss precluded primary treatment of hard tissues, or when grafts were needed, these were done secondarily (24%). Secondary graft procedures involved: block grafts (12%), block grafts secured to a reconstruction plate (3%), and cortiocancellous iliac bone placed into titanium mesh trays (9%). All grafts were harvested from the anterior iliac crest and placed transcutaneously.There were no bone graft failures.

7.1.4. Clinical course

Initial healing of the flaps was uncomplicated in 76% of the patients. However, postoperative discharge from the suture sites was seen in 24% of the patients. This usually resolved within several weeks using daily irrigation and cleansing of the discharge site. None of the soft-tissue flaps sloughed or developed necrosis. Form and function of the regions reconstructed with soft-tissue usually recovered within one year postoperatively. The esthetic results obtained were acceptable in our cases. None required facial nerve grafting, as only the terminal nerve endings were injured in our cases and functional recovery was good.

8. Discussion

8.1. Timing treatment

Ballistic injuries to the face can have minor or often, devastating consequences. The timing, sequence, and appropriate application of surgical procedures and techniques used for reconstruction and rehabilitation of these injuries, have proved to be influential to the final outcome and esthetic result [19]. The staged sequence of treatment dictating the timing of both hard and soft-tissue treatment are dependent to a large extent on surgical judgment and the general condition of the patient. The selection of the appropriate surgical technique as well as the timing of surgery is important to prevent infection, wound dehiscence, graft rejection, facial deformity and subsequent revisional operations. Complications prolong hospital stay, postoperative morbidity and increase treatment costs.

8.2. Basic surgical stages

Surgical management of maxillofacial ballistic wounds has generally been divided into three stages [19,23,24]:

1.   Debridement, fracture stabilization, and primary closure

2.   Reconstruction of hard-tissues, provided that the soft-tissue coverage is adequate (Figure 11).

3.   Rehabilitation of the oral vestibule, alveolar ridge, and secondary correction of residual deformities.

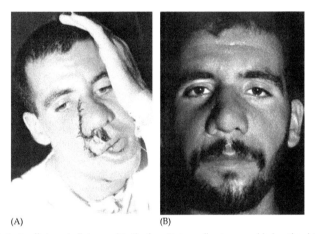

(A)   (B)

Figure 11. (A) Patient suffering a bullet wound to the face. Note small entry wound below the chin and large exit wound through the face. The patients wounds had been closed and a tracheostomy had been performed prior to transfer. The mandible, maxilla, zygoma and nasal bone were fractured. The wound was re-opened, debrided, arch bars were placed and open reduction was done; then the wound was closed. (B) Patient 6 months postoperatively. No other subsequent surgical treatment was necessary.

Often, stages one and two can be done in the first operation [2,7,19]. Early definitive and comprehensive treatment of the facial injury is the mainstay of treatment when indicated. This results in lower morbidity and better results [2,7,19,23-29]. Local undermining and use of regional soft-tissue advancement rotation flaps for primary closure of maxillofacial soft-tissue defects from projectile injuries have proved beneficial from an esthetic and functional point of view [19]. Leaving defects open results in extensive scarring of the facial tissues complicating subsequent surgical procedures and should be avoided [23,24]. Debridement, cleansing and loose closure of locally transferred tissue is a better alternative. Surprisingly, despite the contaminated nature of ballistic injuries of the face, entry and exit wounds of the soft-tissues can be closed primarily following careful debridement and extensive irrigation [19,23,24]. Owing to the excellent facial blood supply, primary closure of facial ballistic wounds is the treatment of choice when indications are met [19,23-25]. Underlying compound facial fractures(without extensive comminution) can be reduced, immobilized and fixed in occlusion at the time of primary closure provided that soft tissue coverage is adequate and soft tissue attachments to the bone are preserved [16,19]. In selected patients without severe comminution or infection, osteosynthesis of all free and attached bone fragments using plates in accordance with AO-ASIF can be performed concomitantly with debridement and primary closure. In such cases it is wise to preserve periosteal blood supply and muscle attachments to the attached bony fragments during reduction and fixation. Antibiotic therapy also plays a major role in the prevention of infection of both hard and soft-tissues after primary closure; early and appropriate surgical debridement, copious irrigation, fixation and immobilization of injured hard tissues, detailed wound closure, drainage, and maintenance of clean dressings, nutrition, and circulating fluid volume are equally important [16,19,23]. The hemodynamics of the patient require correction to optimize oxygen carrying capacity influential in wound healing and prevention of infection in victims who have suffered extensive blood loss [14,16,19,23,24].

8.3. Revisions

In the next stage when facial soft-tissue injuries are treated electively, previous scars should be excised. In order to treat residual defects, the basic surgical strategy should be to try and rearrange the scars to lie in the natural skin folds (Figure 12).

Such revisions and secondary operations are often necessary and were undertaken in 48% of our patients. This involves operations directed towards rehabilitation and re-establishment of a more normal facial appearance and function which include minor cosmetic procedures and scar revisions. Those most commonly indicated are periorbital, around the alar base, the oral commissures and the vermilion border of the lips. Symmetry in these areas is essential. Many of these operations may be performed under local anesthesia and sedation on outpatients. Masticatory rehabilitation and restoration of occlusion is facilitated with osseointegrated implants. The main problem encountered by the surgeon treating facial soft-tissue injuries in victims remains the lack of adequate suitable tissue to close or reconstruct the defects. In the face, muscle function of the reconstructed facial soft tissues, especially in the lips and perioral regions require composite skin-muscle-mucosal flaps, which become reinnervated and show a high degree of functional recovery yielding acceptable results [15-17,21,26].

8.4. Basic flap principles

8.4.1. Patterns

Most local flaps are random pattern flaps with no specific named vascular supply. Examples include rhomboid flaps, V-Y flaps, bilobed flaps and Z-plasty.The length to width ratio of a local flap is very important, and should be approximately 1:1 in most cases to ensure adequate vascular supply to the flap. This ratio is somewhat variable depending on the underlying

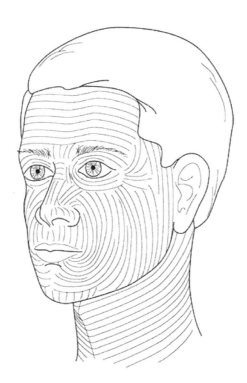

Figure 12. Langer's lines of the face.

vascularity. For example, flaps in highly vascular areas such as the face can be longer with a narrower base, while a poorly vascularized area such as the lower extremity requires that flap length be equal to flap width. Closure of the donor site for a local flap is usually done in two layers: a layer of absorbable deep dermal fine sutures followed by skin closure with intradermal absorbable or transcutaneous monofilament suture. If the sutures are tied too tightly or left in too long, suture marks will be visible, decreasing the esthetic result. When utilized on the face, sutures should be removed in three to seven days. Local flaps remain erythematous and edematous for many weeks, not taking their final form for three to six months or more, thus any revisional operations should wait [27,28].

8.4.2. Defect size assessment

Assessment of defect size is important in planning reconstruction especially in the area of the lips. However, in many cases, assessment of the exact size of the defect can only be done after debridement, approximation of the wound edges and muscles, and when the remaining tissues have been brought into proper position. In patients with scarring, such scar tissue must first be released. When Abbe flaps are contemplated, it should be noted that the flap pedicle should lie directly opposite the defect. The pedicle is based on the labial artery, located 0.5 cm beneath the mucosal lining of the inner aspect of the lip and must be preserved. In designing this flap; the horizontal dimension of the base of the flap along the vermilion, should be one half of the horizontal defect in the upper lip. In all cases, the vertical dimension of the flap and the defect in the upper lip should be equal. It is advocated that the flap should not exceed 2 cm in width so that the lower (donor) lip does not become too constricted [21,26-28]. Division of the pedicle is usually performed after 2-3 weeks.

A common error when using flaps, is the tendency to inadequately mobilize or extend the flaps. All flaps should be of adequate size to remain in place without tension, otherwise dehiscence, scarring, ectropion or increased scleral show may result. On the whole, we feel that, local flaps in the form of lateral flaps, cheek flaps, nasolabial flaps, rotation advancement flaps alone or in combination with Abbe flaps, tissue rearrangement procedures, supporting flaps, or lengthening procedures such as V-Y or Z plasties, are easier to undertake and have less morbidity for the injured patient when compared with distant flaps.

8.4.3. Benefits of the rhomboid flap

The rhomboid flap is versatile and can be used to cover the bullet entry wound (Figure 13).

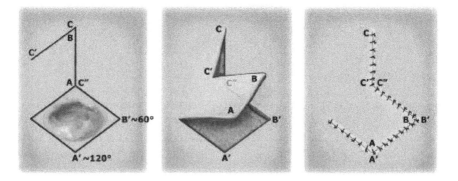

Figure 13. The rhomboid flap can be used to cover the bullet entry wound.

8.4.4. Benefits of Z-plasty

The primary reasons to perform a Z-plasty are to improve contour, release scar contracture, relieve skin tension, and mobilize tissue for reconstructive surgery.

Z-plasty has several main tissue effects:

• Redirection of scar - The new scar reorients from the axis of the central limb to a line connecting the tips of the lateral limbs. Z-plasty is used to redirect the scar into "relaxed skin tension lines" (ie, Langer's lines Figure 12), natural skin folds, or along the border of an esthetic unit (ie, nasolabial fold) to improve cosmetic or functional outcome.

- Lengthening of the scar - Z-plasty lengthens the initial wound or scar. It is used to release contractures and redirect scars (Figure 14).

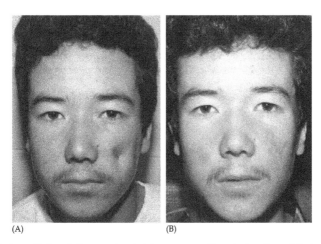

(A)   (B)

Figure 14. (A) Patient suffering a bullet wound to the left zygoma, maxilla and palate. Treated via dermal flaps and Z-plasty. (B)Patient months postoperatively. The Caldwell procedure plus antrostomy was done simultaneously with the soft tissue repair.

The amount of lengthening is related to the angle between the central and lateral limbs. Larger angles produce the most lengthening, but can be difficult to close because of skin tension. Narrow angles (<45°) are easier to close, but produce minimal lengthening and have a higher risk of flap necrosis due to their precarious blood supply.

Central/lateral limb angle	30°	45°	60°	75°	90°
Theoretical gain in length	25%	50%	75%	100%	120%

The 60 degree Z-plasty (ie, classic Z-plasty) is most commonly used because it provides the optimal balance between lengthening and ease of closure.

- Tissue mobilization - Z-plasty mobilizes adjacent tissue to close skin defects that might otherwise have required a skin graft.

8.4.5. Free flaps

Distant or free flaps are not contraindicated and definitely have their place in the treatment and reconstruction of facial defects, and we have used them effectively in many patients. However, we prefer to consider them secondarily or as a final resort, preserving them for failed patients or patients requiring extensive reconstruction of both hard and soft tissues of the face not amenable to local flaps, or for patients with scarred, or ischemic tissues unsuitable for the application of local flaps.

Application of local tissue transfer procedures yield acceptable tissue form, texture, and color match, especially when these procedures are used in combination, and tailored to fit the individual defect moreover, application of these procedures is relatively easy and postoperative morbidity is limited, provided the general condition of the patient is stable, the surgical techniques used have good indications and general flap principles (blood supply, length, size, adequate pedicle and mobilization etc.) have been applied. Form and function of the soft-tissue reconstructed regions usually recover within one year postoperatively. The esthetic results obtained are usually favourable. If the terminal branches of the facial nerve are injured they usually recover (in our cases functional recovery was good).

Author details

Mohammad Hosein Kalantar Motamedi[1], Seyed Hossein Mortazavi[2], Hossein Behnia[2], Masoud Yaghmaei[2], Abbas Khodayari[3], Fahimeh Akhlaghi[3], Mohammad Ghasem Shams[3] and Rashid Zargar Marandi[4]

1 Professor of Oral and Maxillofacial Surgery, Trauma Research Center, Baqiyatallah University of Medical Sciences, and Attending Surgeon, Azad University of Medical Sciences, Tehran, Iran

2 Professor of Oral and Maxillofacial Surgery, Department of Oral and Maxillofacial Surgery, Taleghani Medical Center, Shahid Beheshti University of Medical Sciences, Tehran, Iran

3 Associate Professor of Oral and Maxillofacial Surgery, Department of Oral and Maxillofacial Surgery, Taleghani Medical Center, Shahid Beheshti University of Medical Sciences, Tehran, Iran

4 Neurosurgeon, Department of Neurosurgery, Baqiyatallah University of Medical Sciences. Tehran, Iran

References

[1] Weider, L, Hughes, K, Ciarochi, J, & Dunn, E. Early versus delayed repair of facial fractures in the multiply injured patient. Am Surg (1999). , 65, 790-7.

[2] Motamedi, M. H. Primary treatment of penetrating injuries to the face. J Oral Maxillofac Surg (2007). , 65, 1215-8.

[3] Glapa, M, Kourie, J. F, Doll, D, & Degiannis, E. Early management of gunshot injuries to the face in civilian practice. World J Surg (2007). , 31, 2104-10.

[4] Kincaid, B, & Schmitz, J. P. Tissue injury and healing. Oral Maxillofac Surg Clin North Am (2005). , 17, 241-50.

[5] Ueeck, B. A. Penetrating injuries to the face: Delayed versus primary treatment-considerations for delayed treatment. J Oral Maxillofac Surg (2007). , 65, 1209-14.

[6] Shvyrkov, M. B. Primary surgical treatment of gunshot wounds of facial skeleton. Stomatologiia (Mosk) (2001). , 80, 36-40.

[7] Motamedi, M. H. Primary management of maxillofacial hard and soft tissue gunshot and shrapnel injuries.J Oral Maxillofac Surg. (2003). Dec;, 61(12), 1390-8.

[8] Mclean, J. N, Moore, C. E, & Yellin, S. A. Gunshot wounds to the face-acute management. Facial Plast Surg (2005). , 21, 191-8.

[9] Hollier, L, Grantcharova, E. P, & Kattash, M. Facial gunshot wounds: A 4-year experience. J Oral Maxillofac Surg (2001). , 59, 277-83.

[10] Baig, M. A. Current trends in the management of maxillofacial trauma. Ann R Australas Coll Dent Surg (2002). , 16, 123-7.

[11] Lieblich, S. E, & Topazian, R. G. Infection in the patient with maxillofacial trauma. In: Fonseca RJ, Walker RV, editors. Oral and maxillofacial trauma.Philadelphia: Saunders; (1991). , 1157-1159.

[12] Peleg, M, & Sawatari, Y. Management of gunshot wounds to the mandible.J Craniofac Surg. (2010). Jul;, 21(4), 1252-6.

[13] Vayvada, H, Menderes, A, Yilmaz, M, Mola, F, Kzlkaya, A, & Atabey, A. Management of close-range, high-energy shotgun and rifle wounds to the face. J Craniofac Surg (2005). , 16, 794-804.

[14] Motamedi, M. H, & Behnia, H. Experience with regional flaps in the comprehensive treatment of maxillofacial soft-tissue injuries in warfare victims. J Craniomaxillofac Surg (1999). , 27, 256-9.

[15] Motamedi, M. H, Khatami, S. M, & Tarighi, P. Assessment of severity, causes, and outcomes of hospitalized trauma patients at a major trauma center.J Trauma. (2009). Feb;, 66(2), 516-8.

[16] Motamedi, M. H. Management of firearm injuries to the facial skeleton: Outcomes from early primary intervention. J Emerg Trauma Shock (2011). , 4, 212-6.

[17] Motamedi, M. H, Sagafinia, M, & Famouri-hosseinizadeh, M. Oral and maxillofacial injuries in civilians during training at military garrisons: prevalence and causes.Oral Surg Oral Med Oral Pathol Oral Radiol Endod. (2012). jul:114(1):49-51

[18] Sali Bukhari SG Khan I, Pasha B, Ahmad W. Management of facial gunshot wounds. J Coll Physicians Surg Pak (2010). , 20, 382-5.

[19] Behnia, H. Motamedi MHK: Reconstruction and rehabilitation of short-range, high-velocity gunshot injury to the lower face. J Cranio Maxillofac Surg (1997). , 25, 220-4.

[20] Motamedi, M. H, Hashemi, H. M, Shams, M. G, & Nejad, A. N. Rehabilitation of war-injured patients with implants: analysis of 442 implants placed during a 6-year period. J Oral Maxillofac Surg. (1999). Aug;discussion 914-5., 57(8), 907-13.

[21] Wei-Yung YIH Howerton DW: A regional approach to reconstruction of the upper lip. J Oral Maxillofac Surg (1997).

[22] Taher AA: Management of weapon injuries to the craniofacial skeletonJ Craniofac Surg 9, 371, (1998).

[23] Osborne, T. E. Bays RA: Pathophysiology and management of gunshot wounds to the face: In: Fonseca R J, Walker RV (eds.):Oral and maxillofacial trauma, Philadelphia: WB Saunders, 672, (1991). , 2

[24] Berlin, R, Gerlin, L. E, Jenson, B, et al. Local effects of assault rifle bullets in live tissues. Acta Chir Scand Suppl (1976).

[25] Shelton DW: Gunshot woundsIn: Peterson LJ, Indresano AT, Marciani RD, Roser SM (eds.): Principles of oral and maxillofacial surgery, Philadelphia: JB Lippincott, 596, (1992). , 1

[26] Converse, J. M. Wood-Smith D: Techniques for the repair of defects of the lips and cheeks: In: Converse JM (ed.): Reconstructive Plastic Surgery, Philadelphia: WB Saunders, (1977). , 3, 1547.

[27] Carray, J. H. Vincent MP: Reconstruction of eyelid deformities: In: Georgiade NG, Georgiade GS, Riefkohl R (eds.): Essentials of plastic, maxillofacial and reconstructive surgery. Baltimore, Maryland: Williams and Wilkins, (1987). , 480.

[28] Jackson IT: Local flaps in head and neck reconstructionSt Louis: CV Mosby, 189, (1985).

[29] Kalantar Motamedi MH Comprehensive Management of Maxillofacial Projectile Injuries at the First Operation; "Picking up the Pieces". Trauma Mon. (2013). , 17(4), 365-6.

Cleft Lip and Palate Surgery

Koroush Taheri Talesh and
Mohammad Hosein Kalantar Motamedi

Additional information is available at the end of the chapter

1. Introduction

The treatment of cleft lip and palate deformities requires thoughtful consideration of the anatomic complexies of the deformity and the delicate balance between intervention and growth. Comprehensive and coordinated care from infancy through adolescence is essential in order to achieve an ideal outcome, and surgeons with formal training and experience in all of the phases of care must be actively involved in the planning and treatment. Specific goals of surgical care for children born with cleft lip and palate include the following:

- Normalized esthetics of the lip and nose

- Intact primary and secondary palate

- Normal speech, language, and hearing

- Nasal airway patency

- Class I occlusion with normal masticatory function

- Good dental and periodontal health

- Normal psychosocial development

Successful management of the child born with a cleft lip and palate requires coordinated care provided by a number of different specialties including oral/maxillofacial surgery, otolaryngology, genetics, speech pathology, orthodontics, prosthodontics, and others. In most cases care of patients with congenital clefts has become a subspecialty area of clinical practice within these different professions. In addition to surgery for cleft repair, treatment plans routinely involve multiple treatment interventions to achieve the above-stated goals. Because care is provided over the entire course of the child's development, long-term follow-up is critical under the care of these different health care providers. The formation of interdisciplinary cleft palate teams has served two key objectives of successful cleft care: [1] coordinated care provided by all of the necessary disciplines, and [2] continuity of care with close interval follow-up of the patient throughout periods of active growth and ongoing stages of reconstruction. The best outcomes are achieved when the team's care is centered on the patient, family, and community rather than a particular surgeon, specialty, or hospital. The idea of having an objective team that does not revolve around the desires of one particular individual or discipline is sometimes impeded by competitive interactions between surgical specialties. Historic battles over surgical domains between surgical specialties and economic factors contribute to these conflicts and negatively affect the work of the team. Healthy team dynamic and optimal patient care are achieved when all members are active participants, when team protocols and referral patterns are equitable and based on the surgeons' formal training and experience instead of specialty identity, and when the needs of the child are placed above the needs of the team. [1-3]

2. Prevalence and classification

The occurrence of oral clefts in the United States has been estimated as 1 in 700 births.' Clefts exhibit interesting racial predilections, occurring less frequently in blacks but more so in Asians. Boys are affected by orofacial clefts more often than girls, by a ratio of 3:2. Cleft lip and palate (together) occurs about twice as often in boys as in girls, whereas isolated clefts of the palate (without cleft lip) occur slightly more often in girls. Oral clefts commonly affect the lip, alveolar ridge, and hard and soft palates. Three fourths are unilateral deformities; one fourth are bilateral. The left side is involved more frequently than the right when the defect is unilateral. The cleft may be incomplete, that is, it may not extend the entire distance from lip to soft palate. cleft palate may occur without clefting of the lip. A useful classification divides the anatomy into primary and secondary palates. The primary palate involves those structures anterior to the incisive foramen-the lip and alveolus; the secondary palate consists of those structures posterior to the incisive foramen-the hard and soft palates. Thus an individual may have clefting of the primary palate, the secondary palate, or both.Clefts of the lip may range from a minute notch on the edge of the vermilion border to a wide cleft that extends into the nasal cavity and thus divides the nasal floor. Clefts of the soft palate may also show wide variations from a bifid uvula to a wide inoperable cleft. The bifid uvula is the most minor form of cleft palate, in which only the uvula is clefted. Submucosal clefts of the soft palate are occasionally seen. These clefts are also called occult clefts, because they are not readily seen on cursory examination. The defect in such a cleft is a lack of continuity in the musculature of the soft palate. However, the nasal and oral mucosa is continuous and covers the muscular defect. To diagnose such a defect, the dentist inspects the soft palate while the patient says "ah".This action lifts the soft palate, and in individuals with submucosal palatal clefts, a furrow in the midline is seen where the muscular discontinuity is present. The dentist can also palpate the posterior aspect of the hard palate to detect the absence of the posterior nasal spine, which

is characteristically absent in submucosal clefts. If a patient shows hypernasal speech without an obvious soft palatal cleft, the dentist should suspect a submucosal cleft of the soft palate.[4]

3. Embryology

From an anatomic standpoint the cleft surgeon must have an appreciation for the failure of embryogenesis that results in clefting. There are critical points in the development of the fetus when the fusion of various prominences creates continuity and form to the lip, nose, and palate. Anomalies occur when the normal developmental process is disturbed between these components. Each of these prominences is made up of ectomesenchyme derived from neural crest tissue of the mesencephalon and rhombencephalon. Mesoderm is also present within these prominences as mesenchymal tissue. The prescribed destiny of each of these cells and tissues is controlled by various genes to alter the migration, development, and apoptosis and form the normal facial tissues of the fetus. At the molecular level there are many interdependent factors such as signal transduction, mechanical stress, and growth factor production that affect the development of these tissues. Currently only portions of this complex interplay of growth, development, and apoptosis are clear. At approximately 6 weeks of human embryologic development the median nasal prominence fuses with the lateral nasal prominences and maxillary prominences to form the base of the nose, nostrils, and upper lip. The confluence of these anterior components becomes the primary palate. When this mechanism fails, clefts of the lips and/or maxilla occur. At approximately 8 weeks the palatal shelves elevate and fuse with the septum to form the intact secondary palate. When one palatal shelf fails to fuse with the other components, then a unilateral cleft of the secondary palate occurs. If both of the palatal shelves fail to fuse with each other and the midline septum, then a bilateral cleft of the palate occurs. Fusion occurs when programmed cell death (apoptosis) occurs at the edges of the palatal shelves. The ectodermal component disintegrates and the mesenchyme fuses to form the intact palate. Soon after this the anterior primary palate fuses with the secondary palate and ossification occurs. At any point, if failure of fusion occurs with any of the above components, a cleft will occur of the primary and/or secondary palates. Clefts may be complete or incomplete based on the degree of this failure of fusion.[5-7]

4. Treatment of cleft lip and palate

The aim of treatment of cleft lip and palate is to correct the cleft and associated problems surgically and thus hide the anomaly so that patients can lead normal lives. This correction involves surgically producing a face that does not attract attention, a vocal apparatus that permits intelligible speech, and a dentition that allows optimal function and esthetics. Operations begin early in life and may continue for several years. In view of the gross distortion of tissues surrounding the cleft, it is amazing that success is ever achieved. However, with modern anesthetic techniques, excellent pediatric care centers, and surgeons who have had a wealth of experience because of the frequency of the cleft deformity, acceptable results are commonplace.[3]

5. Timing of surgical repair

The timing of the surgical repair has been and remains one of the most debated issues among surgeons, speech pathologists, audiologists, and orthodontists. It is tempting to correct all of the defects as soon as the baby is able to withstand the surgical procedure. The parents of a child born with a facial cleft would certainly desire this mode of treatment, eliminating all of the baby's clefts as early in life as possible. Indeed the cleft lip is usually corrected as early as possible. Most surgeons adhere to the proven "rule of 10" as determining when an otherwise healthy baby is fit for surgery (i.e., 10 weeks of age, 10 lb in body weight, and at least 10 g of hemoglobin per deciliter of blood). However, because surgical correction of the cleft is an elective procedure, if any other medical condition jeopardizes the health of the baby, the cleft surgery is postponed until medical risks are minimal.[8]

Although different cleft teams time the surgical repair differently, a widely accepted principle is compromise.The lip is corrected as early as is medically possible. The soft palatal cleft is closed between 8 and 18 months of age, depending upon a host of factors. Closure of the lip as early as possible is advantageous, because it performs a favorable "molding" action on the distorted alveolus. It also assists the child in feeding and is of psychologic benefit. The palatal cleft is closed next, to produce a functional velopharyngeal mechanism when or before speech skills are developing. The hard palatal cleft is occasionally not repaired at the time of soft palate repair, especially if the cleft is wide. In such cases, the hard palate cleft is left open as long as possible so that maxillary growth will proceed as unimpeded as possible (Fig. 1). [8]

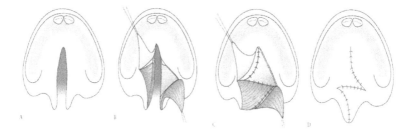

Figure 1. A, Cleft of the secondary palate (both hard and soft) from the incisive foramen to the uvula. B, Furlow double-opposing Z-plasty technique ; Z-plasty flaps developed on the oral and then nasal side. Note the cutbacks creating the nasal side flaps highlighted in blue. C, The flaps are then transposed to lengthen the soft palate. A nasal side closure is completed in the standard fashion anterior to the junction of the hard and soft palate. Generally this junction is the highest area of tension and can be difficult to close. This contributes to the higher fistula rate in this type of repair. D, The oral side flaps are then transposed and closed in a similar fashion completing the palate closure.

Closure of the hard palatal cleft can be postponed at least until all of the deciduous dentition has erupted. This postponement facilitates the use of orthodontic appliances and allows more maxillary growth to occur before scarring from the surgery is induced. Because a significant portion of maxillary growth has already occurred by ages 4 to 5, closure of the hard palate at this time is usually performed before the child's enrollment in school. Removable palatal obturators can be fitted and worn in the meantime to partition the oral and nasal cavities (Table 1).[8]

Staged Reconstruction of Cleft Lip and Palate Deformities	
Procedure	Timing
Cleft lip repair	After 10 weeks
Cleft palate repair	9–18 months
Pharyngeal flap or pharyngoplasty	3–5 years or later based on speech development
Maxillary/alveolar reconstruction with bone grafting	6–9 years based on dental development
Cleft orthognathic surgery	14–16 years in girls, 16–18 years in boys
Cleft rhinoplasty	After age 5 years but preferably at skeletal maturity; after orthognathic surgery when possible
Cleft lip revision	Anytime once initial remodeling and scar maturation is complete but best performed after age 5 years

Table 1. Staged reconstruction of cleft lip and palate deformities

6. Cleft lip and palate repair

6.1. Presurgical taping and presurgical orthopedics

Facial taping with elastic devices is used for application of selective external pressure and may allow for improvement of lip and nasal position prior to the lip repair procedure. In the authors' opinions these techniques often have greater impact in cases of wide bilateral cleft lip and palate where manipulation of the premaxillary segment may make primary repair technically easier. Although one of the basic surgical tenets of wound repair is to close wounds under minimal tension, attempts at improving the arrangement of the segments using taping methods have not shown a measurable improvement. Some surgeons prefer presurgical orthopedic (PSO) appliances rather than lip taping to achieve the same goals.PSO appliances are composed of a custom-made acrylic base plate that provides improved anchorage in the molding of lip, nasal, and alveolar structures during the presurgical phase of treatment. PSOs also add significant cost and time to treatment early in the child's life. Many appliances require a general anesthetic for the initial impression used to fabricate the device. Frequent appointments are necessary for monitoring of the anatomic changes and periodic appliance adjustment.[9-12]

7. Cheilorrhaphy

Cheilorrhaphy is the surgical correction of the cleft lip deformity. The cleft of the upper lip disrupts the important circumoral orbicularis oris musculature. The lack of continuity of this muscle allows the developing parts of the maxilla to grow in an uncoordinated manner so that the cleft in the alveolus is accentuated. At birth the alveolar process on the unaffected side may appear to protrude from the mouth. The lack of sphincteric muscle control from the orbicularis oris will cause a bilateral cleft lip to exhibit a premaxilla that protrudes from the base of the nose and produces an unsightly appearance. Thus restoration of this muscular sphincter with lip repair has a favorable effect on the developing alveolar segments.[8]

8. Unilateral cleft lip repair

Clefts of the lip and nose that are unilateral present with a high degree of variability, and thus each repair design is unique. The basic premise of the repair is to create a three-layered closure of skin, muscle, and mucosa that approximates normal tissue and excises hypoplastic tissue at the cleft margins. Critical in the process is the reconstruction of the orbicularis oris musculature into a continuous sphincter. The Millard rotation-advancement technique has the advantage of allowing for each of the incision lines to fall within the natural contours of the lip and nose. This is an advantage because it is difficult to achieve "mirror image" symmetry in the unilateral cleft lip and nose with the normal side immediately adjacent to the surgical site A Z-plasty technique such as the Randall-Tennison repair may not achieve this level of symmetry because the Z-shaped scar is directly adjacent to the linear non-clefted philtrum. Achieving symmetry is more difficult when the rotation portion of the cleft is short in comparison to the advancement segment. Primary nasal reconstruction may be considered at the time of lip repair to reposition the displaced lower lateral cartilages and alar tissues. Several techniques are advocated, and considerable variation exists with respect to the exact nasal reconstruction performed by each surgeon. The primary nasal repair may be achieved by releasing the alar base, augmenting the area with allogeneic subdermal grafts, or even a formal open rhinoplasty (Fig. 2).[13-15]

9. Bilateral lip repair

Bilateral cleft lip repair can be one of the most challenging technical procedures performed in children with clefts. The lack of quality tissue present and the widely displaced segments are major challenges to achieving exceptional results, but superior technique and adequate

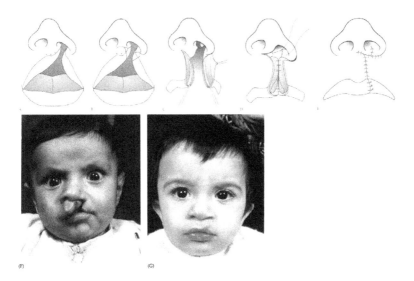

Figure 2. A, Complete unilateral cleft of the lip highlighting the hypoplastic tissue in the cleft site that is not used in the reconstruction. Nasal deformities are typical in the unilateral cleft, including displaced lower lateral nasal cartilages, deviated anterior septum, and nasal floor clefting. B, The typical markings for the authors' preferred repair are shown highlighting the need to excise the hypoplastic tissue and approximate good vermilion and white roll tissue for the repair. C, Once the hypoplastic tissue has been excised, the three layers of tissue are dissected (skin, muscle, and mucosa). It is important to completely free the orbicularis oris from its abnormal insertions on the anterior nasal spine area and lateral alar base. Nasal flaps are also incorporated into the dissection to repair the nasal floor (not shown). D, The orbicularis oris muscle is approximated with multiple interrupted sutures, and the vermilion border/white roll complex is reconstructed. The nasal floor and mucosal flaps are approximated. E, The lateral flap is advanced and the medial segment is rotated downward to create a healing scarline that will resemble the natural philtral column on the opposite side. The incision lines are hidden in natural contours and folds of the nose and lip. F, Four month-old boy with complete unilateral cleft lip and severe step maxillary segment.G, Lip closure was done by Millard II technique.

mobilization of the tissue flaps usually yields excellent esthetic results.Additionally the columella may be quite short in length, and the premaxillary segment may be significantly rotated. Adequate mobilization of the segments and attention to the details of only using appropriately developed tissue will yield excellent results even in the face of significant asymmetry. Some surgeons have used aggressive techniques to surgically lengthen the columella and preserve hypoplastic tissue using banked fork flaps.Early and aggressive tissue flaps in the nostril and columella areas do not look natural after significant growth has occurred and result in abnormal tissue contours. While surgical attempts at lengthening the columella may look good initially, they frequently look abnormally long and excessively angular later in life (Fig. 3).[16]

In severe cleft lip with protruded premaxilla early closure of the cleft and aligning of orbicularis oris muscle and return of lip sphinctric function ultimately cause setbacking of the premaxilla reducing the alveolar cleft gap and step and facilitate anterior palate and alveolar cleft repair (Fig. 4).

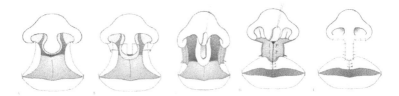

Figure 3. A, Complete bilateral cleft of the lip and maxilla showing hypoplastic tissue along the cleft edges. The importance of the nasal deformity is evident in the shorter columella and disrupted nasal complexes. B, Markings of the authors' preferred repair are shown with emphasis on excision of hypoplastic tissue and approximating more normal tissue with the advancement flaps. C, A new philtrum is created by excising the lateral hypoplastic tissue and elevating the philtrum superiorly. Additionally the lateral advancement flaps are dissected into three distinct layers (skin, muscle, and mucosa). Nasal floor reconstruction is also performed. D, The orbicularis oris musculature is approximated in the midline with multiple interrupted and/or mattress sutures. This is critical in the total reconstruction of the functional lip. There is no musculature present in the premaxillary segment, and this must be brought to the midline from each lateral advancement flap. The nasal floor flaps are sutured at this time as well. The new vermillion border is reconstructed in the midline with good white-roll tissue advanced from the lateral flaps. E, Final approximation of the skin and mucosal tissues is performed leaving the healing incision lines in natural contours of the lip and nose.

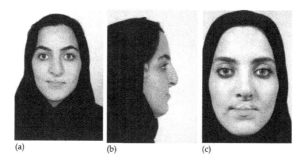

(a)   (b)   (c)

Figure 4. A, 20 year-old girl with severe bilateral cleft lip and alveolar cleft with protruded premaxilla. B, After early closure of cleft lip with Veau's technique the protruded premaxilla was corrected.C, After closed Rhinoplasty and columella lengthening.

10. Palatorrhaphy

Palatorrhaphy is usually performed in one operation, but occasionally it is performed in two.In two operation the soft palate closure is usually performed first and the hard palate closure is performed second. The primary purpose of the cleft palate repair is to create a mechanism capable of speech and deglutition without significantly interfering with subsequent maxillary growth. Thus creation of a competent velopharyngeal mechanism and partitioning of the nasal and oral cavities are prerequisites to achieving these goals. The aim is to obtain a long and mobile soft palate capable of producing normal speech. Extensive stripping of soft tissues from bone will create more scar formation.The exact timing of repair of a palate cleft is controversial.

Generally the velum must be closed prior to the development of speech sounds that require an intact palate. On average this level of speech production is observed by about 18 months of age in the normally developing child. If the repair is completed after this time, compensatory speech articulations may result.Repair completed prior to this time allows for the intact velum to close effectively,appropriately separating the nasopharynx from the orophayrynx during certain speech sounds. When repair of the palate is performed between 9 and 18 months of age,the incidence of associated growth restriction affecting the maxillary development is approximately 25%.If repair is carried out earlier than 9 months of age,then severe growth restriction requiring future orthognathic surgery is seen with greater frequency. At the same time proceeding with palatoplasty prior to 9 months of age is not associated with any increased benefit in terms of speech development so the result is an increase in growth related problems with an absence of any functional benefit.Using only the chronologic age it seems that carrying out the operation during the 9 to 18 months timeline best balances the need to address functional concerns such as speech development with the potential negative impact on growth. Many techniques have been described for repair of the palate.The Bardach two-flap palatoplasty uses two large full-thickness flaps that are mobilized with layered dissection and brought to the midline for closure.This technique preserves the palatal neurovascular bundle as well as a lateral pedicle for adequate blood supply. The von Langenbeck technique is similar to the Bardach palatoplasty but preserves an anterior pedicle for increased blood supply to the flaps. This technique is also successful in achieving a layered closure but may be more difficult when suturing the nasal mucosa near the anteriorly based pedicle attachments.The authors do not favor push-back techniques as they may incur more palatal scarring, restrict growth, and do not show ameasurable benefit in speech.Another common technique is the Furlow double-opposing Z plasty,which attempts to lengthen the palate by taking advantage of a Z-plasty technique on both he nasal mucosa and the oral mucosa.This technique can be effective at closing the palate but has been reported by some to have a higher rate of fistula formation at the junction of the softand hard palates where theoretical lengthening of the soft palate may compromise the closure (Fig 5).[17-19]

11. Alveolar cleft grafts

The alveolar cleft defect is usually not corrected in the original surgical correction of either the cleft lip or the cleft palate. As a result, the cleft-afflicted individual may have residual oronasal fistulae in this area, and the maxillary alveolus will not be continuous because of the cleft. Because of this, five problems commonly occur: [1] oral fluids escape into the nasal cavity, [2] nasal secretion drains into the oral cavity, [3] teeth erupt into the alveolar cleft, [4] the alveolar segments collapse, and [5] if the cleft is large, speech is adversely affected. Alveolar cleft bone grafts provide several advantages: First, they unite the alveolar segments and help prevent collapse and constriction of the dental arch, which is especially important if the maxilla has been orthodontically expanded. Second, alveolar cleft bone grafts provide bone support for teeth adjacent to the cleft and for those that will erupt into the area of the cleft. Frequently, the bone support on the distal aspect of the central incisor is thin, and the height of the bone support

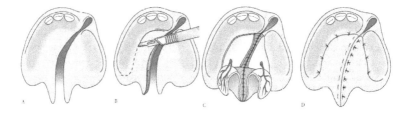

Figure 5. A, Unilateral cleft of the primary and secondary palates with typical involvement from the anterior vestibule to the uvula. B, Bardach palatoplasty technique requires two large full-thickness mucoperiosteal flaps to be elevated from each palate shelf. The anterior portion(anterior to the incisive foramen) of the cleft is not reconstructed until the mixed dentition stage.C, A layered closure is performed in the Bardach palatoplasty by reapproximating the nasal mucosa. The muscle bellies of the levator palatini are elevated off of their abnormal insertions on the posterior palate. They are then reapproximated in the midline to create a dynamic functional sling for speech purposes. D, Once the nasal mucosa and musculature of the soft palate are approximated, the oral mucosa is closed in the midline. The lateral releasing incisions are quite easily closed primarily due to the length gained from the depth of the palate. In rare cases, in very wide clefts a portion of the lateral incisions may remain open and granulate by secondary intention.

varies. These teeth may show slight mobility because of this lack of bone support. Increasing the amount of alveolar bone for this tooth will help ensure its periodontal maintenance. The canine tends to erupt into the Cleft site and, with healthy bone placed into the cleft will maintain good periodontal support during eruption and thereafter. The third benefit of alveolar cleft grafts is closure of the oronasal fistula, which will partition the oral and nasal cavities and prevent escape of fluids between them.[20]

Cleft management should always involve a multidisciplinary team, with the expertise to develop a proper treatment plan. Difficulties may arise when the priorities of one specialty compete with those of another. If the surgical team is faced with an orthodontic provider who feels strongly that it is appropriate to align the maxillary central incisors as soon as they erupt, it will be necessary for the alveolar defect to be grafted earlier to prevent compromise of osseous support for the central incisors. Some orthodontists and surgeons believe that palatal expansion is necessary prior to grafting. These teams may find that it is more appropriate to graft patients at a later age, as it may take months to achieve the desired expansion prior to the graft.

12. Source of bone graft

The selection of the ideal grafting material is somewhat dependent on the timing of the graft. In primary bone grafting, the rib is the only site for adequate quantity of bone with acceptable morbidity. In the mixed dentition stage, the rib is not as appropriate as other sites such as the calvaria or iliac crest. These options would also be possible sources for bone for late secondary grafting, as well as grafts from the mandibular symphysis and possibly the tibia.

13. Iliac crest

Potential advantages of the iliac crest bone graft include low morbidity and high volume of viable osteoblastic cells (cancellous bone); two teams may work simultaneously, and this procedure is well accepted by the patient.

14. Allogeneic bone and bone substitutes

In an effort to eliminate the morbidity and time necessary to harvest bone from any autogenous site, some authors have evaluated allogeneic bone as a potential source of graft material. Studies have shown that allogeneic bone can be used successfully to graft secondary alveolar cleft defects and that results can be compared favorably with those achieved with autogenous bone. However, the demands of bone healing in the alveolar defect where there is potential communication between the graft and the nasal and oral cavity may make this less predictable in large cleft defects or bilateral clefts. In general, bone healing with autogenous bone is biologically different than with allogeneic bone. Autogenous bone grafts initiate an angioblastic response early in the healing process, and some of the transplanted cells remain viable, resulting in a more rapid formation of new bone. In contrast, allogeneic bone grafts demonstrate slower revascularization, as there are no viable cells transferred with the graft. In summary, autogenous bone harvested from the iliac crest remains the most predictable technique.[21]

15. Surgical technique for grafting the cleft alveolus

The ideal technique will meet the following criteria:

1. Predictable closure of the nasal floor produces a watertight barrier between the graft and the nasal cavity

2. Access to closure of residual palatal and labial fistula

3. Keratinized attached tissue is maintained around the teeth adjacent to the cleft and at the site where the yet unerupted lateral incisor and canine will erupt

4. Mobilization of tissue is adequate to close large defects without tension, when such defects are present

5. The vestibule is not shortened, and scarring is not excessive

Given these requirements, the technique most often used employs advancing buccal gingival and palatal flaps. This approach has some disadvantages, including the following:

1. Difficulty obtaining closure in large bilateral clefts, which heal by secondary intention of full-thickness wounds created by the advancement

2. A four-corner suture line that approximates the flaps directly overlying the graft, which may lead to dehiscence

3. The possibility that elevating large full thickness mucoperiosteal flaps leads to growth alteration in young patients.However, when compared with finger flaps and trapezoidal flaps, which can shorten the vestibule and placenonkeratinized tissue around the dentition, this approach remains the best.[21]

In our center we prefer harvesting bone graft orally from the symphysis or anterior border of ramus without changing patient position because of easy access and the rate of success is comparable to other methods.

Author details

Koroush Taheri Talesh[1] and Mohammad Hosein Kalantar Motamedi[2]

1 Oral and Maxillofacial Surgery Tabriz University of Medical Sciences and Azad University of Medical Sciences,Tehran, Iran

2 Oral and Maxillofacial Surgery Baqiyatallah University of Medical Sciences Trauma Research Center,Tehran, Iran

References

[1] Costello, B. J, Ruiz, R. L, & Turvey, T. Surgical management of velopharyngeal insufficiency in the cleft patient. In: Oral and maxillofacial surgery clinics of North America: secondary cleft surgery. Philadelphia (PA): W.B. Saunders; (2002). , 539-551.

[2] Ruiz, R. L, Costello, B. J, & Turvey, T. Orthognathic surgery in the cleft patient. In: Ogle O, editor.Oral and maxillofacial surgery clinics of North America: secondary cleft surgery.Philadelphia (PA): W.B. Saunders; (2002). , 491-507.

[3] Costello, B. J, Shand, J, & Ruiz, R. L. Craniofacial and orthognathic surgery in the growing patient. Selected Readings Oral Maxillofacial Surg (2003). , 11(5), 1-20.

[4] Tolarova, M. M, & Cervenka, J. Classification and birth prevalence of orofacial clefts. Am J Med Genet (1998). , 75, 126-37.

[5] Tolarova, M. Etiology of clefts of lip and/or palate: 23 years of genetic follow-up in 3660 individual cases. In: Pfeifer G, editor. Craniofacial abnormalities and clefts of the lip,alveolus, and palate. Stuttgart: Thieme;(1991). , 16-23.

[6] Gorlin, R, Cohen, M. J, & Levin, L. Syndromes of the head and neck. 4th ed. New York (NY):Oxford University Press; (2003). orofacial clefting. Cleft lip and palate: a physiological approach, Oral Maxillofac Clin North Am 2000;, 12, 379-97.

[7] Shaikh, D, Mercer, N. S, Sohan, K, et al. Prenatal diagnosis of cleft lip and palate. Br J PlastSurg (2001). , 54, 288-9.

[8] Posnick, J. C. The staging of cleft lip and palate reconstruction: infancy through adolescence.In: Posnick JC, editor. Craniofacial and maxillofacial surgery in children and young adults. Philadelphia (PA):W.B. Saunders;(2000). , 785-826.

[9] Poole, R, & Farnworth, T. K. Preoperative lip taping in the cleft lip. Ann Plast Surg (1994). , 32, 243-9.

[10] Shaw, W. C, & Semb, G. Current approaches to the orthodontic management of cleft lip and palate. J R Soc Med (1990). , 83, 30-3.

[11] Ross, R. B. MacNamera MC. Effect of presurgical infant orthopedics on facial esthetics in complete bilateral cleft lip and palate. Cleft Palate Craniofac J (1994). , 31, 68-73.

[12] Grayson, B. H, Santiago, P. E, Brecht, L. E, et al. Presurgical nasoalveolar molding in infants with cleft lip and palate. Cleft Palate Craniofac J (1999). , 36, 486-98.

[13] Randall, P. Long-term results with the triangular flap technique for unilateral cleft lip repair. In: Bardach J, Morris H, editors. Multidisciplinary management of cleft lip and palate. Philadelphia (PA): W.B. Saunders;(1990). , 173.

[14] Millard, D. R. Cleft craft: the evolution of its surgery. Alveolar and palatal deformities. Boston (MA): Little Brown; (1980). , 3

[15] Posnick, J. C. Cleft-orthognathic surgery: the unilateral cleft lip and palate deformity. In:Posnick JC, editor. Craniofacial and maxillofacial surgery in children and young adults. Philadelphia (PA): W.B. Saunders;(2000). , 860-907.

[16] Posnick, J. C. Cleft-orthognathic surgery: the bilateral cleft lip and palate deformity. In: Posnick JC, editor. Craniofacial and maxillofacial surgery in children and young adults. Philadelphia (PA): W.B. Saunders;(2000). , 908-950.

[17] Posnick, J. C. Cleft-orthognathic surgery: the isolated palate deformity. In:Posnick JC, editor. Craniofacial and maxillofacial surgery in children and young adults. Philadelphia (PA): W.B. Saunders; (2000). , 951-978.

[18] Posnick, J. C, & Tompson, B. Cleft-orthognathic surgery. Complications and long-term results. Plast Reconstr Surg (1995).

[19] Dorf, D. S, & Curtin, J. W. Early cleft palate repair and speech outcome: a ten year experience. In: Bardach J,Morris HI..Multidisciplinary management of cleft lip and palate.Philadelphia (PA): W.B. Saunders; (1990). , 341-348.

[20] Sindet-pedersen, S, & Enemark, H. Reconstruction of alveolar clefts with mandibular or iliac crest bone graft: a comparative study. JOral Maxillofac Surg (1990). , 48, 554-8.

[21] Sadove, A. M, Nelson, C. L, Eppley, B. L, et al. An evaluation of calvarial and iliac donor sites in alveolar cleft grafting. Cleft Palate J (1990). , 27, 225-8.

Chapter 8

Current Advances in Mandibular Condyle Reconstruction

Tarek El-Bialy and Adel Alhadlaq

Additional information is available at the end of the chapter

1. Introduction

The temporomandibular joint, like any other synovial joint, can be the subject of severe degenerative pathological conditions as well as fracture and ankylosis. Advanced conditions may require rib or hip grafts, allografts, or total joint replacement. All current approaches suffer from inherent shortcomings and the search continues for a new approach to reconstruct the mandibular condyle with minimal or no side effects. Stem cell-based tissue engineering approach to reconstruct the mandibular condyle has long been introduced; however its potential clinical application requires long and costly dedicated research programs. Other therapeutic physical approaches to enhance tissue regenerative capacity have also been proposed, however their potential application needs further attention and investigation.

2. Clinical indication

Articular joints have a poor innate ability to regenerate following either injury or disease. Among these diseases that affect articular joints is arthritis. In Canada, arthritis is the leading cause of work disability, with an economic cost of $4.4 billion in 1998 alone [1]. Statistics Canada reports estimated that 6 million Canadians will suffer from some form of arthritis by 2026, a significant increase from the current prevalence of four million Canadians [2]. The temporomandibular joint (TMJ) connects the mandible to the skull and is vital for speech, chewing, and swallowing.It is comprised of a mandibular condyle and an articular disk. TMJ is susceptible to arthritis, fractures, ankylosis, and dysfunctional syndromes that affect over 10 million individuals in North America [3-9]. To date, artificial joint replacement is considered the standard therapeutic procedure for degenerated TMJ, but this treatment approach has a high cost and non-predictive outcome [10]. According to the Canadian Joint Replacement Registry, a total of 97,671 patients had different joint replacements between years 2007-2010 [11].It has been reported that about 10% showed foreign body response to TMJ metal replacement with allergic reaction to metal [12]. Consequently, developing effective methods to replace articular condyle are of paramount importance to current/modern society. This book chapter discusses in detail contemporary methods and future directions of mandibular condylar reconstruction.

3. Mesenchymal stem cells

Mesenchymal stem cells (MSCs) are increasingly being used in joint tissue engineering research [13-19]. Tissue engineering ofmandibular condyle as a whole has been proposed in the literature; however an in-vivo utilization of this technique is in need of further investigation based upon compelling evidence from pilot data [15-22]. Some limitations to MSCs based therapy include the extended time needed in the laboratory to expand them and differentiate them into chondrogenic and osteogenic lineages. An improved approach to enhance the expansion and differentiation of MSCs is highly demanded. Also, understanding MSCs differentiation process and their characterization must be achieved before they can be used safely and effectively in articular joint replacement.

The current approach used to tissue engineer articular constructs involves conditioning with some type of mechanical stress. Existing mechanical conditioning techniques to enhance engineered tissues are in the form of bioreactors, BioFlex mechanical modulation technologies (Flexercell), and Instron machines. However, these approaches are short of clinical application should the engineered tissue require more mechanical modulation after in-vivo implantation for functional use.

4. Low intensity pulsed ultrasound

Low intensity pulsed ultrasound (LIPUS) therapy stimulates stem cell growth and differentiation [20,23-24]. We have shown in a pilot study in rabbits that LIPUS may enhance tissue engineered mandibular condyles. This compelling preliminary data needs to be validated in a statistically determined study design. Moreover, there is increasing supporting data in the literature that the stimulatory effect of LIPUS on cell expansion and differentiation is dose dependent. The LIPUS is considered the preferred method of mechanical stimulation, also known as "preferred bioreactor" [25].

5. Articular condyle

An articular condyle consists of articular cartilage and subchondral bone (Fig. 1) [20]. Despite a common developmental origin from mesenchyme, the articular cartilage and subchondral bone have two distinct adult tissue phenotypes with few common morphological features. However, both tissues are structurally integrated and function in harmony to withstand mechanical loading up to several times the body's weight [26].

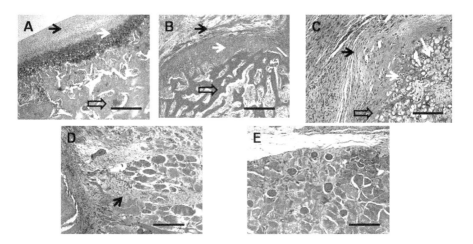

Figure 1. Photomicrographs of the histological examination of normal condyle showing fibrocartilage (black arrow) hypertrophic zone (white arrow) and subchondoral bone (hollow arrow) (Bar =100 μm)[20].

In osteochondral defects, bone regeneration can readily occur in the presence of an adequate blood supply up to a certain bony defect size. In contrast, articular cartilage has a poor capacity for self-regeneration. Furthermore, once articular cartilage is damaged, it undergoes degenerative events such as loss and/or destruction of key structural components, including type II collagen and proteoglycans. The poor capacity of cartilage for self-regeneration is likely attributed to the paucity of tissue-forming cells (i.e., chondrocytes) [27] and the lack of access to systemically available mesenchymal stem cells because the cartilage tissue is avascular. Thus, the self-regenerating capacity of articular cartilage is limited due to the sparsely available chondroprogenitor cells and/or the scant local mesenchymal stem cells that are habitual residents. Importantly, the articular cartilage is devoid of a nerve supply. Thus, articular cartilage injuries are often not accompanied by joint pain until the damage has progressed to involve the subchondral bone, which contains rich nerve supply [28]. In many of these disorders, structural damage of the TMJ necessitates surgical replacement.

6. TMJ replacement

The current TMJ replacement techniques utilize bone/cartilage grafts, muscles and artificial materials [9, 29-30]. Despite certain level of reported clinical success, autografts are associated with donor site morbidity such as discomfort in ambulation, sensorial loss over the donor region, scars, and contour deformity when bone is harvested from the iliac bone. Also, predictability of clinical outcome of autografts is reported to be substandard with graft overgrowth in 10% of patients and undergrowth in 57% of patients, and a relatively high incidence of re-operation with 23% of patients requiring re-grafting [31-34].Alternatively, alloplastic and xenoplastic grafts are associated with potential transmission of pathogens and immunorejection [35-37].The failure rate of using alloplastic grafts to reconstruct the TMJ has been reported to reach 30% [38]. To date, there is no consistent clinically-effective and safe method to replace the TMJ or mandibular condyle.

7. Biological replacement of mandibular condyle

Biological replacement efforts for reconstruction of the mandibular/articular condyles have included using osteoblasts and chondroblasts/chondrogenic cells from different tissue/cell sources [15-22,38-41]. However, these efforts have been limited by several obstacles including: a) scarcity of stem cells with the capacity to differentiate into chondrogenic and osteogenic cells, b) different bone ingrowth patterns [37], c) different rates of the scaffold degradation compared to matrix production [15], and d) inferior mechanical properties of the regenerative tissue for clinical use [40]. Moreover, the integration of tissue engineered constructs for osteochondral repair requires an inordinate amount of time (3-6 months in rabbit femur heads [21],6-12 months in horses [41], and up to 9 months in sheep [19]). Regeneration of articular joints utilizing a cell-free scaffold by cell homing to the area shows some success [18]. However, this process did not provide full articular condyle replacement. In addition, this proof of principle lasted 9 weeks to obtain some articular joint regeneration in rabbits, which translates to 9 to 12 months in humans, given the difference in metabolism between the two species [42]. This lengthy time of manipulation can be complicated by tissue culture problems such as infection. Another attempt to tissue engineer mandibular condyle using porcine stem cells demonstrated bone formation in-vitro; however there was no attempt or success in translating this technique into in-vivo utilization [43]. A similar recent study demonstrated the possibility of tissue engineering a complete mandibular condyle in-vitro; however in-vivo utilization of this technique has yet to be studied[44]. Interestingly, this study highlighted the importance of bioreactor in stem cell expansion and differentiation [44]. It was first reported that tissue engineered osteochondral constructs from MSCs can be shaped into human-size mandibular condyles while maintaining the shape and size after extended period of in-vivo implantation [15,17,18]. Not only these constructs demonstrate MSCs-driven formation of osteochondral tissue-like histologically, but also both tissue types showed good histological integration attributed to the use of the same scaffolding material in both layers, and thus avoiding the potential fibrous tissue infiltration between the two layers usually observed in composite constructs [15,17,18].Our team was the first to report on the possibility of engineering condyles from stem cells [15,17,18] (Figure 2).

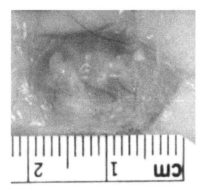

Figure 2. Appearance of a tissue engineered osteochondral construct holding the shape and dimensions of a human mandibular condyle during harvest after 12 weeks of subcutaneous implantation in the dorsum of immunodeficient mouse.

Although most of the recent studies, including ours, are focused on engineering scaffolds in the shape of mandibular or articular condyles [15,17,18,44], future research is needed to implement tissue engineered condyles into clinical application and to demonstrate functional integration. It is well known that inadequate mechanical strength is considered a major impediment to cartilage tissue engineering [45,46]. The material properties of tissue-engineered cartilage constructs are in the range of kilopascals [47], which are orders of magnitude lower than normal articular cartilage (in the range of megapascals) [48-53]. Different techniques have attempted to improve the quality of tissue-engineered articular joints. Pulsed electromagnetic fields (PEMF) have been shown to increase chondrocyte and osteoblast-like cell proliferation [54,55]. Bioreactors including LIPUS enhance the material properties of tissue-engineered cartilage constructs [25,56,57]. Cyclic compressive loading induces phenotypic changes in cartilaginous and osseous tissues in cell culture, scaffolds, and in-vivo [58-70]. Also, mechanical stimulation enhances the expression of vascular endothelial growth factor (VEGF) which is important for angiogenesis and bone formation in the mandibular condyles [71]. These important discoveries support the potential for clinical application of different forms of mechanical stimulation to enhance tissue-engineered joint tissues.

8. Low intensity pulsed ultrasound (LIPUS)

Low intensity pulsed ultrasound (LIPUS) is a form of mechanical stimulation that has been used to enhance healing of fractured bone and other tissues. Details about the current literature and the potential use of LIPUS for better autologous stem cell based mandibular condyle (ASCMC) will be discussed below. It is clear that there is a vital need for an approach to enhance stem cell expansion and differentiation for tissue engineering of articular condyles. LIPUS can be an effective tool to enhance tissue-engineering of mandibular condyles for many reasons.

Importantly, LIPUS is the preferred method of mechanical stimulation, also reported as "preferred bioreactor" [25] as it enhances angiogenesis [20, 72-76].This is especially relevant because vasculature is required to integrate the engineered tissue with the native surrounding tissues [77]. Recent studies showed that LIPUS enhances stem cell expansion and differentiation in tissue culture [78,79]. Also, LIPUS has been shown to enhance periosteal cell expansion [79] and stimulate bone marrow stem cells (BMSCs) expansion and differentiation into chondrogenic lineage [78,80-83].The matrix production and proliferation of the intervertebral disc cells in culture has been shown to be enhance by LIPUS [82]. In addition, LIPUS enhances osteoblast matrix formation [796,83] and minimizes apoptosis of human stem cells in-vitro [84]. The optimum LIPUS application time in bone fracture healing has been identified [85]; however, the optimum LIPUS treatment timing in articular condyle replacement is yet to be studied.Despite recent studies that have shown that the stimulatory effect of LIPUS in tissue culture is dose-dependent (treatment time) [23,24,75,78,86-88], the use of LIPUS has not resulted in any severe adverse events in tissue culture [88], human or animal models [89-92]. Our research has demonstrated that LIPUS can enhance stem cell expansion in monolayers [20-23-24] (Figure 3).There was an increase in cell number after LIPUS application for 20 minutes per day for 3 weeks. A future projectcan aim to optimize using LIPUS to enhance cell proliferation to a significant level that may justify its routine use in tissue engineering.

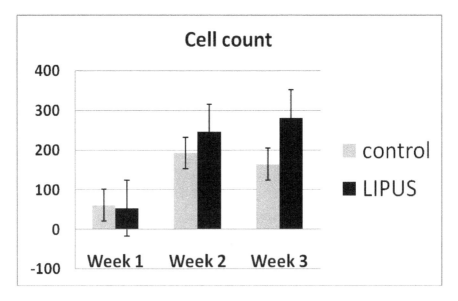

Figure 3. Rat BMSC count after treatment with 20 minutes per day for three weeks.It can be seen that LIPUS enhances cell count compared to untreated BMSCs by (20 minutes per day for three weeks). This reflects that LIPUS stimulates BMSC expansion and this stimulatory effect is treatment time-dependent. This experiment was performed three times and the presented data represents the average and standard error of nine samples [three trials in triplicate]. There is a significant difference in cell number at week 3 between the control and LIPUS treated BMSCs (P<0.05) [23].

In addition, LIPUS enhances expression of bone morphogenetic proteins from pluripotent cells [88]. Moreover, we have shown that LIPUS application for 20 minutes per day for 4 weeks increased the expression of collagen II and osteopontin expression in osteogenic-induced differentiation of stem cells (P<0.05)[Figure 4 and Table A] [20].

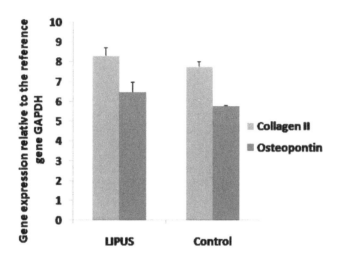

Figure 4. qPCR results of LIPUS treated (20 minutes/day) osteogenic differentiated BMSCs for four weeks and controls. LIPUS treated osteogenic cells expressed more osteopontin and collagen type II genes (normalized to GAPDH) which is indicative of enhancing osteogenic differentiation of BMSCs affected by LIPUS. Both graphs represent results of performing qPCR on nine samples (three trials in triplicate). This increase in Collagen II and Osteopontin by LIPUS is statistically significant (P< 0.005)[20].

Gene of interest	Average + Standard deviation		P
	LIPUS	Control	
Collagen II	8.3 + 0.4	6.4 + 0.5	0.009*
Osteopontin	7.7 + 0.02	5.7 + 0.3	0.004*

Table 1. Collagen II and osteopontin gene expression in vitro as evaluated by qPCR. Gene expression is presented as percentage to the reference gene GAPDH. Non parametric analysis (Mann-Whitney U) shows a statistical significant increase in Collagen II and Osteopontin gene expression by LIPUS when compared to non LIPUS treated samples [20].

Also, LIPUS application to gingival stem cells statistically increased the gene expression of alkaline phosphatase (ALP) in tissue culture (Figure 5) [88].

Figure 5. Alkaline phosphatase (ALP) gene expression was increased by daily treatment of GFs with 10 minutes LIPUS for 4 weeks as evaluated by qPCR. Data represents average of five replicates with the error bar representing standard deviation [885].

Our preliminary data indicated that LIPUS application enhanced osteogenic and chondrogenic differentiation of bone marrow stem cells in collagen sponges in-vitro (Figure 6) as determined by histochemical staining (safranin O for chondrogenic differentiation and von Kossa staining for osteogenic differentiation) [20].

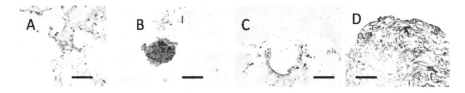

Figure 5. In-vitro chondrogenesis and osteogenesis of BMSCs in samples of collagen scaffolds. A: Positive reaction to safranin O (red staining) of BMSC-derived chondrogenic cell chondrogenic tissue formation in the control [no LIPUS] scaffolds following four-week treatment with chondrogenic medium, B: Increased (red staining) positive reaction to safranin O of the BMSC-derived chondrogenic cells treated with LIPUS and chondrogenic medium for four weeks. C: Positive but weak reaction to Von Kossa silver staining (black staining) of BMSC-derived osteogenic cells in the control [no LIPUS] scaffolds following four-week treatment with osteogenic medium. D: Increased positive reaction to Von Kossa silver staining (black staining) of the BMSC-derived chondrogenic cells treated with LIPUS treatment and osteogenic medium for four weeks. More mineralization nodules are observed with LIPUS treatment. Bar is 100 μm [20].

Finally, we have shown that LIPUS enhances tissue-engineered mandibular condyles in a pilot study invivo [20](Figures 7-13). This was confirmed qualitatively by MicroCT scanning, histological evaluations (safranin O and Von Kossa staining) (Figures 9-12) as well as quantitatively by histomorphometric analysis (Figure 13).

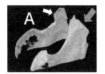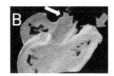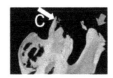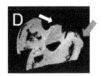

Figure 6. MicroCT scanning of: (A) Group 1 (TEMC + LIPUS); (B) Group 2 (TEMC no LIPUS) (C) Group 3 (scaffold with no cells + LIPUS) and (D) scaffold with no cells and with no LIPUS. In each rabbit, the yellow arrow refers to normal condyle and the white arrow refers to the experimental site (either TEMC or empty scaffold). It can be seen that LIPUS enhanced TEMC as indicated by close morphology of the LIPUS-assisted TEMC compared to the normal condyle (A). The condylar healing was not as pronounced when there were cells present in the scaffold but no LIPUS was applied (B). LIPUS did enhance some healing of the amputated condyle site even without a scaffold (C). The negative control (empty scaffold and no LIPUS) showed no signs of healing (D). Note: TEMC consisted of a scaffold and chondrogenic and osteogenic cells [20].

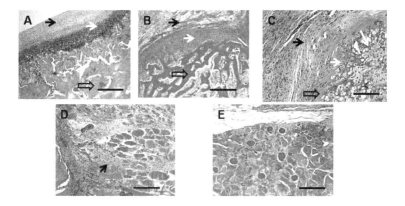

Figure 7. Photomicrographs of the histological examination of (A) normal condyle; (B) LIPUS-assisted TEMC in group 1; (C) TEMC with no LIPUS; (D) empty scaffold with LIPUS; and (E) empty scaffold without LIPUS. The LIPUS-enhanced TEMC (B) has comparable histological features to the normal condyle (A), and TEMC without LIPUS (C) shows some structural integration between the chondrogenic and osteogenic parts of the TEMCs. The empty scaffolds (D, E) show inflammatory cell invasion without bone or cartilage formation. Black arrows refer to fibrocartilage area, white arrows refer to condylarcartilage or new cartilage formed by TEMC areas, and empty arrows refer to condylar bone or new bone formed by the TEMC. Scale bar: 100 mm [20].

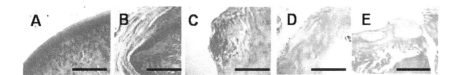

Figure 8. Photomicrographs of safranin O stained histological slides of (A) normal condyle; (B) LIPUS assisted TEMC; (C) TEMC with no LIPUS; (D) Empty scaffold with LIPUS; and (E) empty scaffold without LIPUS. It can be seen that the cartilaginous part of the normal condyle and TEMC have comparable safranin O staining that indicates improved chondrogenesis with LIPUS compared to either empty scaffolds (D and E). TEMC with no LIPUS still shows some reaction to safranin O staining but not like TEMC and LIPUS (Magnification = 16 X) [20].

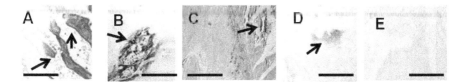

Figure 9. Photomicrographs of Von Kossa stained histological slides of (A) Normal condyle; (B) LIPUS assisted TEMC; (C) TEMC with no LIPUS; (D) Empty scaffold with LIPUS and (F) Empty scaffold without LIPUS.LIPUS assisted TEMC and normal condyle show comparable Von Kossa silver staining of the bone underlying the cartilage/chondrogenic part of the condyle/TEMC. In empty scaffold implanted condyles, minimum or no mineralization nodules can be seen by Von Kossa silver staining. Bar is 100 μm [20].

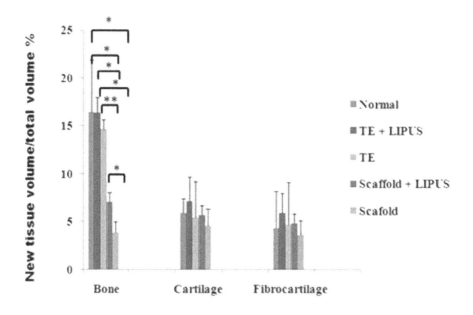

Figure 10. Histomorphomteric Analysis of the TEMC + LIPUS or empty scaffolds + LIPUS [20].

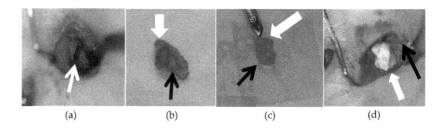

(a)   (b)   (c)   (d)

Figure 11. A: Rabbits after condylectomy [white arrow indicates condylectomy site]. B: Condyle after dissection [white arrow refers to the cartilage part and black arrow refers to the bony part of the condyle], C: Collagen sponge containing chondrogenic [white arrow] and osteogenic [black arrow] cells; D: TEMC [black arrow] fixed in place with white bone cement [white arrow]. (Photos from pilot study [20])

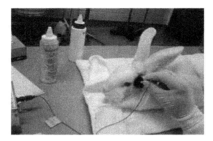

Figure 12. LIPUS: application to the rabbit while it is restrained [20].

8.1. Mechanical stress and intracellular signaling

There is growing evidence in the literature that integrins are promising candidates for sensing extracellular matrix-derived mechanical stimuli and converting them into biochemical signals [93-96]. Integrin-associated signaling pathways include an increase in tyrosine phosphoryla-tion of several signaling proteins, activation of serine/threonine kinases, and alterations in cellular phospholipid and calcium levels [97-98]. These events are associated with the forma-tion of focal adhesions, which contain structural proteins such as Src, and Shc. Focal adhesions act as a bridge to link integrin cytoplasmic domain to the cytoskeleton and activate integrin-associated signaling pathways, such as the mitogen-activated protein kinase (MAPK) pathway [99] and the Rho pathway [100-101]. Rho and its downstream target Rho kinase/Rho-associated coiled-coil-containing protein kinase (ROCK) [102] are involved in the reorganization of cytoskeletal components [99], [102-103]. It has been recently reported that β1 integrin plays predominant roles for shear-induced signaling and gene expression in osteoblast-like MG63 cells on FN, COL1, and Laminin (LM) and that $\alpha v\beta 3$ also plays significant roles for such responses in cells on fibronectin (FN). The β1 integrin-Shc association leads to the activation of ERK, which is critical for shear induction of bone formation-related genes in osteoblast-like cells [103]. Moreover, $\alpha 5\beta 1$ integrin is expressed by chondrocytes [104] and it plays an important role in mechanically enhanced cartilage tissue engineering. Furthermore, integrins were found to be responsible for ultrasound-induced cell proliferation. It has been suggested that integrins act as mechanotransducers to transmit acoustic pulsed energy into intracellular biochemical signals inducing cell proliferation [105]. It has been reported recently that LIPUS activates the phosphatidylinositol 3 kinase/Akt pathway and stimulates the growth of chondrocytes [106] as well as increases FAK, ERK-1/2, and IRS-1 expression of intact rat bone cells [107]. This has yet to be investigated in MSC derived chondrocytes and in osteoblasts-like cells.

9. Conclusion

The literature supports that mechanical stress, for example LIPUS have a stimulatory effect on stem cell expansion and differentiation as well as enhancing stem cell matrix production in-vitro and in a pilot study in-vivo in rabbits. However, these results need to be validated in a large scale in-vivo.We are now poised to prove these effects in a large scale study. Although the optimum mechanical stimulation, for example LIPUS treatment time, for bone fracture healing is well documented, the corollary for enhancing autologous stem cell based replacement of mandibular condyles has not been investigated. This represents a major gap of knowledge in the field of tissue engineering considering the numerous positive utilizations of mechanical stimulation as well as LIPUS reported in the literature. Overall, the current literature and knowledge developed through our and others' research has the potential to increase our understanding of the details of LIPUS induced chondrogenesis and osteogenesis and how to utilize LIPUS to enhance articular joint replacement using MSCs. Furthermore, this knowledge could give rise to a novel cell-based therapy for replacement of mandibular condyles as well as other tissue types.

Acknowledgements

This work is sponsored by King Saud University, Riyadh, Saudi Arabia

Author details

Tarek El-Bialy[1*] and Adel Alhadlaq[2]

*Address all correspondence to: telbialy@ualberta.ca; aalhadlaq@hotmail.com

1 Faculty of Medicine and Dentistry, 7-020D Katz Group Centre for Pharmacy and Health Research, University of Alberta, Edmonton, Alberta, Canada

2 College of Dentistry, King Saud University, Riyadh, Saudi Arabia

References

[1] Health C. Health Canada; Economic Impact of Illness in Canada. Ottawa: Public Works and Government Services Canada.Catalogue # H21-136/1998E, 2002. 1998. Ref Type: Internet Communication

[2] Statistics C. Canadian Community Health Survey (CCHS). Public Health Agency of Canada http:,www.phac-aspc.gc.ca/publicat/ac/ac_3e-eng.php, editors. 2000. Ref Type: Internet Communication.

[3] Ribeiro RF, Tallents RH, Katzberg RW, Murphy WC, Moss ME, Magalhaes AC, Tavano O. The prevalence of disc displacement in symptomatic and asymptomatic volunteers aged 6 to 25 years. J Orofac Pain 11:37-47, 1997.

[4] Ferrari R, Leonard MS. Whiplash and temporomandibular disorders: a critical review. J Am Dent Assoc 129:1739-1745,1998.

[5] Israel HA, Diamond B, Saed-Nejad F, Ratcliffe A. Osteoarthritis and synovitis as major pathoses of the temporomandibular joint: comparison of clinical diagnosis with arthroscopic morphology. J Oral Maxillofac Surg 56:1023-1027, 1998.

[6] Sano T, Westesson PL, Larheim TA, Rubin SJ, Tallents RH. Osteoarthritis and abnormal bone marrow of the mandibular condyle. Oral Surg Oral Med Oral Pathol Oral RadiolEndod 87:243-252, 1999.

[7] Stohler CS (1999) Muscle-related temporomandibular disorders. J Orofac Pain 13:273-284,1999. Goddard G, Karibe H. TMD prevalence in rural and urban Native American populations. Cranio 20:125-128, 2002.

[8] Bell RB, Blakey GH, White RP, Hillebrand DG, Molina A. Staged reconstruction of the severely atrophic mandible with autogenous bone graft and endosteal implants. J Oral Maxillofac Surg 60:1135-1141, 2002.

[9] Henning TB, Ellis E 3rd, Carlson DS. Growth of the mandible following replacement of the mandibular condyle with the sternal end of the clavicle: an experimental investigation in Macacamulatta. J Oral Maxillofac Surg 50:1196-1206, 1992.

[10] Westermark A, Koppel D, Leiggener C.: Condylar replacement alone is not sufficient for prosthetic reconstruction of the temporomandibular joint. Int J Oral Maxillofac Surg. 2006 Jun;35(6):488-92.

[11] Data Quality Documentation for Users: Canadian Joint Replacement Registry, 2007–2008 to 2009–2010 Data. http://secure.cihi.ca/cihiweb/products/DQ_CJRR_2007-2010_e.pdf. Ref Type: Internet Communication

[12] Sidebottom AJ, Speculand B, Hensher R.: Foreign body response around total prosthetic metal-on-metal replacements of the temporomandibular joint in the UK. Br J Oral Maxillofac Surg. 2008 Jun;46(4):288-92.

[13] Chen FH, Tuan RS. Mesenchymal stem cells in arthritic diseases. Arthritis Res Ther. 2008;10:223-235.

[14] Goldring MB. Are bone morphogenetic proteins effective inducers of cartilage repair? Ex vivo transduction of muscle-derived stem cells.[comment]. Arthritis & Rheumatism. 2006;54:387-389.

[15] Alhadlaq A, Mao JJ. Tissue-engineered Neogenesis of Human-shaped Mandibular Condyle from Rat Mesenchymal Stem Cells. J Dent Res 82:951-6, 2003.

[16]   Alhadlaq A, Mao JJ. Mesenchymal stem cells: isolation and therapeutics. Stem Cells Dev 13:436-48, 2004.

[17]   Alhadlaq A, Elisseeff J, Hong L, Williams C, Caplan AI, Sharma B, Kopher RA, Tomkoria S, Lennon DP, Lopez A, Mao JJ. Adult stem cell driven genesis of human-shaped articular condyle. Ann Biomed Eng 32:911-923, 2004.

[18]   Alhadlaq A, Mao JJ.: Tissue-engineered osteochondral constructs in the shape of an articular condyle. J Bone Joint Surg Am 87:936-44, 2005.

[19]   Pilliar RM, Kandel RA, Grynpas MD, Zalzal P, Hurtig M.: Osteochondral defect repair using a novel tissue engineering approach: sheep model study. Technol Health Care 15(1):47-56, 2007.

[20]   El-Bialy, T., Uludag, H., Jomha, N., and Badylak, S.: In vivo ultrasound assisted tissue engineered mandibular condyle: a pilot study in rabbits. Tissue Eng Part C Methods (2010 Dec;16(6):1315-23).

[21]   Lee, C.H., Cook, J.L., Mendelson, A., Moioli, E.K., Yao, H., Mao, J.J.: Regeneration of the articular surface of the rabbit synovial joint by cell homing: a proof of concept study. Lancet 376: 440–48, 2010.

[22]   Shao X, Goh JC, Hutmacher DW, Lee EH, Zigang G.: Repair of large articular osteochondral defects using hybrid scaffolds and bone marrow-derived mesenchymal stem cells in a rabbit model. Tissue Eng 12(6):1539-51, 2006.

[23]   Ang, W.T.; Yu,C.; Chen, J.; El-Bialy, T.H.; Doschak, M.; Uludag, H. and Tsui, Y.: System-on-chip Ultrasonic Transducer for Dental Tissue Formation and Stem Cell Growth and Differentiation, Proceeding of the IEEE, May, 2008.

[24]   Aldosary, T.A.; Uludag, H.; Doschak, M.; Chen, J.; Tsui, Y. and EL-Bialy, T.: Effect of Ultrasound on Human Umbilical Cord Perivascular-Stem Cell Expansion. IADR, Toronto, July 2008, Abstract # 873.

[25]   Marvel S, Okrasinski S, Bernacki SH, Loboa E, Dayton PA.: The development and validation of a LIPUS system with preliminary observations of ultrasonic effects on human adult stem cells. IEEE Trans UltrasonFerroelectrFreq Control. 2010 Sep;57(9): 1977-84.

[26]   Martin, RB, Burr DB, and Sharkey NA. Skeletal Tissue Mechanics. New York: Springer-Verlag, 1998.

[27]   Poole AR, Kojima T, Yasuda T, Mwale F, Kobayashi M, Laverty S.: Composition and structure of articular cartilage: a template for tissue repair.Clin Orthop Relat Res. 2001 Oct;(391 Suppl):S26-33.

[28]   LeResche L. Epidemiology of temporomandibular disorders: implications for the investigation of etiologic factors. Crit Rev Oral Biol Med 8:291-305, 1997.

[29] MacIntosh RB. The use of autogenous tissues for temporomandibular joint reconstruction. J Oral MaxillofacSurg 58:63-69, 2000.

[30] Canter HI, Kayikcioglu A, Saglam-Aydinatay B, Kiratli PO, Benli K, Taner T, Erk Y.: Mandibular reconstruction in Goldenhar syndrome using temporalis muscle osteofascial flap. J Craniofac Surg. 2008 Jan;19(1):165-70.

[31] Dodson TB, Bays RA, Pfeffle RC, Barrow DL. Cranial bone graft to reconstruct the mandibular condyle in Macacamulatta. J Oral Maxillofac Surg 55:260-267, 1997.

[32] Wolford LM, Karras SC. Autologous fat transplantation around temporomandibular joint total joint prostheses: preliminary treatment outcomes. J Oral Maxillofac Surg 55:245-251, 1997.

[33] Wan DC, Taub PJ, Allam KA, Perry A, Tabit CJ, Kawamoto HK, Bradley JP. Distraction osteogenesis of costocartilaginous rib grafts and treatment algorithm for severely hypoplastic mandibles. PlastReconstr Surg. 2011 May;127(5):2005-13

[34] Mercuri LG. The use of alloplastic prostheses for temporomandibular joint reconstruction. J Oral Maxillofac Surg 58:70-75, 2000.

[35] Meyer RA. Costal cartilage for treatment of temporomandibular joint ankylosis. PlastReconstr Surg 109:2168-2169, 2002.

[36] van Minnen B, Nauta JM, Vermey A, Bos RR, Roodenburg JL. Long-term functional outcome of mandibular reconstruction with stainless steel AO reconstruction plates. Br J Oral Maxillofac Surg 40:144-148, 2002.

[37] Lindqvist C, Söderholm AL, Hallikainen D, Sjövall L. : Erosion and heterotopicbone formation afteralloplastic temporomandibular joint reconstruction. J Oral Maxillofac Surg. 1992 Sep;50(9):942-9;

[38] Poshusta AK, Anseth KS. Photopolymerized biomaterials for application in the temporomandibular joint. Cells Tissues Organs 169:272-278, 2001.

[39] Springer IN, Fleiner B, Jepsen S, Acil Y. Culture of cells gained from temporomandibular joint cartilage on non -absorbable scaffolds. Biomaterials 22:2569-2577, 2001.

[40] Chu TM, Orton DG, Hollister SJ, Feinberg SE, Halloran JW. Mechanical and in vivo performance of hydroxyapatite implants with controlled architectures. Biomaterials 23:1283-1293, 2002.

[41] Barnewitz D, Endres M, Krüger I, Becker A, Zimmermann J, Wilke I, Ringe J, Sittinger M, Kaps C.: Treatment of articular cartilage defects in horses with polymer-based cartilage tissue engineering grafts. Biomaterials 27(14):2882-9, 2006.

[42] Losken, A.; Mooncy, M.P., and Siegel, M.I.: A comparative study of mandibular growth patterns in seven animal models. J. Oral MAxillofac. Surg., 50: 490-495; 1992.

[43] Abukawa H, Terai H, Hannouche D, Vacanti JP, Kaban LB, Troulis MJ.: Formation of a mandibular condyle in vitro by tissue engineering. J Oral Maxillofac Surg. 2003 Jan; 61(1):94-100.

[44] Grayson WL, Fröhlich M, Yeager K, Bhumiratana S, Chan ME, Cannizzaro C, Wan LQ, Liu XS, Guo XE, Vunjak-Novakovic G. Engineering anatomically shaped human bone grafts.: ProcNatlAcad Sci U S A. 2010 Feb 23;107(8):3299-304. Epub 2009 Oct 9.

[45] Mow VC, Wang CC.: Some bioengineering considerations for tissue engineering of articular cartilage. Clin Orthop Relat Res (367 Suppl):S204-23, 1999.

[46] Sikavitsas VI, Temenoff JS, Mikos AG. Biomaterials and bone mechanotransduction. Biomaterials 22:2581-2593, 2001.

[47] LeBaron RG, Athanasiou KA. Ex vivo synthesis of articular cartilage. Biomaterials 21:2575-2587, 2000.

[48] Patel RV, Mao JJ.: Microstructural and elastic properties of the extracellular matrices of the superficial zone of neonatal articular cartilage by atomic force microscopy. Front Biosci 8:a18-25, 2003.

[49] Cohen B, Chorney GS, Phillips DP, Dick HM, Buckwalter JA, Ratcliffe A, Mow VC. The microstructural tensile properties and biochemical composition of the bovine distal femoral growth plate. J Orthop Res 10:263-275, 1992.

[50] Hu K, Radhakrishnan P, Patel RV, Mao JJ. Regional structural and viscoelastic properties of fibrocartilage upon dynamic nanoindentation of the articular condyle. J Struct Biol 136:46-52, 2001.

[51] Narmoneva DA, Wang JY, Setton LA. Nonuniform swelling-induced residual strains in articular cartilage. J Biomech 32:401-8, 1999.

[52] Clark PA, Rodriguez T, Sumner DR, Clark AM, Mao JJ. Micromechanical analysis of bone-implant interface using atomic force microscopy. Proceedings of BMES-IEEE 16:304-305, 2002.

[53] Goldstein SA. Tissue engineering: functional assessment and clinical outcome. Ann N Y Acad Sci 961:183-192, 2002.

[54] De Mattei M, Caruso A, Pezzetti F, Pellati A, Stabellini G, Sollazzo V, Traina GC.: Effects of pulsed electromagnetic fields on human articular chondrocyte proliferation. Connect Tissue Res. 42:269-79, 2001.

[55] Hartig M, Joos U, Wiesmann HP.: Capacitively coupled electric fields accelerate proliferation of osteoblast-like primary cells and increase bone extracellular matrix formation in vitro. Eur Biophys J. 29:499-506, 2000

[56] Pei M, Solchaga LA, Seidel J, Zeng L, Vunjak-Novakovic G, Caplan AI, Freed LE. Bioreactors mediate the effectiveness of tissue engineering scaffolds. FASEB J 16:1691-1694, 2002.

[57]   Gemmiti CV, Guldberg RE.: Fluid Flow Increases Type II Collagen Deposition and Tensile Mechanical Properties in Bioreactor-Grown Tissue-Engineered Cartilage. Tissue Eng. 12:469-79, 2006.

[58]   Vance J, Galley S, Liu DF, Donahue SW.: Mechanical stimulation of MC3T3 osteoblastic cells in a bone tissue-engineering bioreactor enhances prostaglandin E2 release. Tissue Eng. 11:1832-9, 2005.

[59]   El Haj AJ, Wood MA, Thomas P, Yang Y.: Controlling cell biomechanics in orthopaedic tissue engineering and repair. Pathol Biol (Paris). 53:581-9, 2005.

[60]   Janssen FW, Oostra J, Oorschot A, van BlitterswijkCA.: A perfusion bioreactor system capable of producing clinically relevant volumes of tissue-engineered bone: in vivo bone formation showing proof of concept. Biomaterials. 27:315-23, 2006.

[61]   Stevens MM, Marini RP, Schaefer D, Aronson J, Langer R, Shastri VP.: In vivo engineering of organs: the bone bioreactor. ProcNatlAcad Sci U S A. 9;102:11450-5, 2005.

[62]   Service RF.: Tissue engineering. Technique uses body as 'bioreactor' to grow new bone. Science.309:683, 2005.

[63]   Vunjak-Novakovic G, Meinel L, Altman G, Kaplan D.: Bioreactor cultivation of osteochondral grafts. Orthod Craniofac Res. 8:209-18, 2005.

[64]   Haasper C, Colditz M, Kirsch L, Tschernig T, Viering J, Graubner G, Runtemund A, Zeichen J, Meller R, Glasmacher B, Windhagen H, Krettek C, Hurschler C, Jagodzinski M.: A system for engineering an osteochondral construct in the shape of an articular surface: Preliminary results. Ann Anat. 2008;190(4):351-9. Epub 2008 Mar 18.

[65]   Davisson T, Kunig S, Chen A, Sah R, Ratcliffe A. Static and dynamic compression modulate matrix metabolism in tissue engineered cartilage. J Orthop Res 20:842-848, 2002.

[66]   Mizuno S, Tateishi T, Ushida T, Glowacki J. Hydrostatic fluid pressure enhances matrix synthesis and accumulation by bovine chondrocytes in three-dimensional culture. J Cell Physiol 193:319-327, 2002.

[67]   Elder SH, Goldstein SA, Kimura JH, Soslowsky LJ, Spengler DM. Chondrocyte differentiation is modulated by frequency and duration of cyclic compressive loading. Ann Biomed Eng 29:476-482, 2001.

[68]   Huang CY, Hagar KL, Frost LE, Sun Y, Cheung HS.: Effects of cyclic compressive loading on chondrogenesis of rabbit bone-marrow derived mesenchymal stem cells. Stem Cells. 22:313-23, 2004.

[69]   Butler DL, Juncosa-Melvin N, Boivin GP, Galloway MT, Shearn JT, Gooch C, Awad H. Functional tissue engineering for tendon repair: A multidisciplinary strategy using mesenchymal stem cells, bioscaffolds, and mechanical stimulation. J Orthop Res. 2008 Jan;26(1):1-9

[70] Kinneberg KR, Nirmalanandhan VS, Juncosa-Melvin N, Powell HM, Boyce ST, Shearn JT, Butler DL. Chondroitin-6-sulfate incorporation and mechanical stimulation increase MSC-collagen sponge construct stiffness. J Orthop Res. 2010 Aug;28(8): 1092-9.

[71] Rabie ABM, Shum L, Chayanupatkul A. VEGF and bone formation in the glenoid fossa during forward mandibular positioning.Am J Orthod Dentofacial Orthop. 2002;122:202–209.

[72] Young SR, Dyson M. The effect of therapeutic ultrasound on angiogenesis. Ultrasound Med Biol. 1990;16:261–269.

[73] El-Bialy T, El-Shamy I, Graber TM, Growth modification of the rabbit mandible using therapeutic ultrasound: is it possible to enhance functional appliance results?, Angle Orthod; 73:631-639, 2003.

[74] El-Bialy, T.H., Hassan, A., Albaghdadi, T., Fouad, H.A., and Maimani, A.R., Growth modification of the mandible using Ultrasound in baboons: A preliminary report, Am J Orthod Dentofacial Orthop, 130(4);435e7-14, 2006.

[75] El-Bialy TH, Royston TJ, Magin RL, Evans CA, Zaki Ael-M, Frizzell LA, The effect of pulsed ultrasound on mandibular distraction. Ann Biomed Eng;30:1251-61, 2002.

[76] Peter J. Yang, Johnna S. Temenoff. Engineering Orthopedic Tissue Interfaces. Tissue Eng Part B Rev. 2009 June; 15(2): 127–141.

[77] Yoon JH, Roh EY, Shin S, Jung NH, Song EY, Lee DS, Han KS, Kim JS, Kim BJ, Jeon HW, Yoon KS.: Introducing pulsed low-intensity ultrasound to culturing human umbilical cord-derived mesenchymal stem cells. Biotechnol.Lett. 2009 Mar;31(3):329-335.

[78] Schumann D, Kujat R, Zellner J, Angele MK, Nerlich M, Mayr E, Angele P.: Treatment of human mesenchymal stem cells with pulsed low intensity ultrasound enhances the chondrogenic phenotype in vitro. Biorheology. 2006;43(3-4):431-43.

[79] Leung KS, Cheung WH, Zhang C, Lee KM, Lo HK.: Low intensity pulsed ultrasound stimulates osteogenic activity of human periosteal cells. Clin Orthop Relat Res.(418): 253-9, 2004.

[80] Ebisawa K, Hata K, Okada K, Kimata K, Ueda M, Torii S, Watanabe H.: Ultrasound enhances transforming growth factor beta-mediated chondrocyte differentiation of human mesenchymal stem cells. Tissue Eng. 10(5-6):921-9, 2004.

[81] Cui JH, Park K, Park SR, Min BH.: Effects of low-intensity ultrasound on chondrogenic differentiation of mesenchymal stem cells embedded in polyglycolic acid: an in vivo study. Tissue Eng. 12:75-82, 2006.

[82] Iwashina T, Mochida J, Miyazaki T, Watanabe T, Iwabuchi S, Ando K, Hotta T, Sakai D.: Low-intensity pulsed ultrasound stimulates cell proliferation and proteoglycan

production in rabbit intervertebral disc cells cultured in alginate. Biomaterials. 27:354-61, 2006.

[83] Naruse K, Miyauchi A, Itoman M, Mikuni-Takagaki Y.: Distinct anabolic response of osteoblast to low-intensity pulsed ultrasound. J Bone Miner Res 18:360-9, 2003.

[84] Lee, H.J. Choi, BH, Min, BH and Park, S.R. Low-Intensity Ultrasound Inhibits Apoptosis and Enhances Viability of Human Mesenchymal Stem Cells in Three-Dimensional Alginate Culture During Chondrogenic Differentiation: Tissue Engineering, 13: (5) 1049-1057, 2007.

[85] Tsai CL, Chang WH, Liu TK.: Preliminary studies of duration and intensity of ultrasonic treatments on fracture repair. Chin J Physiol. 1992;35(1):21-6. Erratum in: Chin J Physiol;35:168, 1992.

[86] El-Bialy, T., Hassan, A.H., Alyamani, A. and Albaghdadi, T.: Treatment of Hemifacial Microsomia by therapeutic ultrasound and hybrid functional appliance. A nonsurgical approach. Open Access Journal of Clinical Trials, 2, 29-36, 2010.

[87] Chan CW, Qin L, Lee KM, Cheung WH, Cheng JC, Leung KS.: Dose-dependent effect of low-intensity pulsed ultrasound on callus formation during rapid distraction osteogenesis. J Orthop Res. 2006 Nov;24(11):2072-9.

[88] Mostafa, N.Z.; Uludag, H.; Dederich, D.N.; Doschak, M.R.; El-Bialy, T.H.: Anabolic Effects of Low Intensity Pulsed Ultrasound on Gingival Fibroblasts, Archives of Oral Biology, 54 (8), 7 43 - 7 48, 2009.

[89] Hata T, Aoki S, Manabe A, Hata K, Miyazaki K. Three dimensional ultrasonography in the first trimester of human pregnancy. Hum Reprod 1997;12:1800-4.

[90] Blaas HG, Eik-Nes SH. Advances in the imaging of the embryonic brain. Croat Med J 1998;39:128-31.

[91] Turnbull DH, Foster FS. In vivo ultrasound biomicroscopy in developmental biology. Trends Biotechnol 2002;20:S29-33.

[92] Mende U, Zoller J, Dietz A, Wannenmacher M, Born IA, Maier, H. Ultrasound diagnosis in primary staging of head-neck tumors. Radiologe 1996;36:207-16.

[93] Ingber DE.: Mechanosensation through integrins: cells act locally but think globally. 1: ProcNatlAcad Sci U S A. 2003 Feb 18;100(4):1472-4. Epub 2003 Feb 10.

[94] Giancotti FG, Ruoslahti E.: Integrin signaling. Science. 1999 Aug 13;285(5430): 1028-32.

[95] Aplin AE, Howe A, Alahari SK, Juliano RL.: Signal transduction and signal modulation by cell adhesion receptors: the role of integrins, cadherins, immunoglobulin-cell adhesion molecules, and selectins. Pharmacol Rev. 1998 Jun;50(2):197-263.

[96] Schlaepfer DD, Hunter T.: Integrin signalling and tyrosine phosphorylation: just the FAKs? Trends Cell Biol. 1998 Apr;8(4):151-7.

[97] Riveline D, Zamir E, Balaban NQ, Schwarz US, Ishizaki T, Narumiya S, Kam Z, Geiger B, Bershadsky AD.: Focal contacts as mechanosensors: externally applied local mechanical force induces growth of focal contacts by an mDia1-dependent and ROCK-independent mechanism. J Cell Biol. 2001 Jun 11;153(6):1175-86.

[98] Clark EA, King WG, Brugge JS, Symons M, Hynes RO.: Integrin-mediated signals regulated by members of the rho family of GTPases. J Cell Biol. 1998 Jul 27;142(2): 573-86.

[99] Shyy JY, Chien S.: Role of integrins in cellular responses to mechanical stress and adhesion. CurrOpin Cell Biol. 1997 Oct;9(5):707-13.

[100] Kaibuchi K, Kuroda S, Amano M.: Regulation of the cytoskeleton and cell adhesion by the Rho family GTPases in mammalian cells. Annu Rev Biochem. 1999;68:459-86.

[101] Ridley AJ, Hall A.: The small GTP-binding protein rho regulates the assembly of focal adhesions and actin stress fibers in response to growth factors. Cell. 1992 Aug 7;70(3):389-99.

[102] Hotchin NA, Hall A. The assembly of integrin adhesion complexes requires both extracellular matrix and intracellular rho/racGTPases.J Cell Biol. 1995 Dec;131(6 Pt 2): 1857-65.

[103] Lee DY, Yeh CR, Chang SF, Lee PL, Chien S, Cheng CK, Chiu JJ.: Integrin-mediated expression of bone formation-related genes in osteoblast-like cells in response to fluid shear stress: roles of extracellular matrix, Shc, and mitogen-activated protein kinase.J Bone Miner Res. 2008 Jul;23(7):1140-9.

[104] Takashi Nishida, Harumi Kawaki, Ruth M. Baxter, R. Andrea DeYoung, Masaharu-Takigawa, Karen M. Lyons.: N2 (Connective Tissue Growth Factor) is essential for extracellular matrix production and integrin signaling in chondrocytes. J Cell Commun Signal. 2007 June

[105] Zhou S, Schmelz A, Seufferlein T, Li Y, Zhao J, Bachem MG.: Molecular mechanisms of low intensity pulsed ultrasound in human skin fibroblasts.J Biol Chem. 2004 Dec 24;279(52):54463-9. Epub 2004 Oct 12.

[106] Takeuchi, R., Ryo,A., Komitsu, N., Mikuni-Takagaki, Y., Fukui, A., Takagi, Y., Shiraishi, T., Morishita, S., Yamazaki, Y., Kumagai, K., Aoki, I., Saito,T..: Low-intensity pulsed ultrasound activates the phosphatidylinositol 3 kinase/Akt pathway and stimulates the growth of chondrocytes in three-dimensional cultures: a basic science study. Arthritis Res Ther. 2008; 10(4): R77.

[107] ViníciusBuarque de Gusmão, C., Pauli, J.R., AbdallaSaad,M.J., Alves, J.M., Belangero, W.D.: Low-intensity Ultrasound Increases FAK, ERK-1/2, and IRS-1 Expression of In-

tact Rat Bones in a Noncumulative Manner. Clin Orthop Relat Res. 2010 April; 468(4): 1149–1156.

Chapter 9

The Cosmetic Considerations in Facial Defect Reconstruction

Mazen Almasri

Additional information is available at the end of the chapter

1. Introduction

The 21st century is designated by the era of communication, multimedia, hi-tech gadgets and network connection programs that help people share the news, events, pictures and recent advancements throughout the world. The common denominator is the facial profile or image. Moreover, facial cosmetic advertisement, media, and products are taking big share of this phenomenon. Ad's usually display male and female individuals of variable age groups to assure reflecting the best facial and body figure toward the outer world. This goes hand-in-hand with the humanitarian beauty jealousy, the raised professional standards, the increase of sales managements and marketing business, the application of the quality management protocols in working environment, and the increase in self-satisfaction level and confidence. All the aforementioned issues raise the demand for facial cosmetics surgery and better quality of life. Thus, the new era of maxillofacial reconstruction had upgraded the concepts of management. The oral and maxillofacial surgeon may encounter severe panfacial trauma, severe maxillofacial tumors, abnormal congenital defects and secondary facial deformities that require extreme caution while constructing the surgical treatment plan. Such plan should provide the patient not only with better surgical outcome, but also improve the emotional self-satisfaction, family acceptance, quality of life, and easier re-integration into the working society.

Maxillofacial fractures are still a common cause of hospital admission for treatment all over the world [1,2]. Although major advancements in the safety of motor vehicles and traffic regulations traffic accidents (RTAs); are still a major problem in developing countries while alcohol abuse is the major stimulant associated with personal altercations [3]. It is well proved that most of the facial injuries do occur in the second to fourth decades of life, which is usually a studying or a working period in the individuals' life. Thus, although the concept of reduction and fixation is the main pillar of treating facial fractures, it is still not enough. Facial cosmetics and esthetics are important considerations that merit attention; treatment of the fracture alone is not always enough. Many fracture are associated with facial defects (Figure 1).

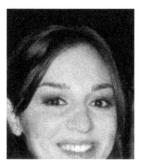

Figure 1. An attractive 26 year- old female treated for a right orbital fracture and fixation through transconjuctival approach with lateral canthotomy. Although the results are very good she still feels that the palpebral fissure space on the right eye is smaller than the left eye. (Special gratitude to my colleague Dr E. Elizabeth, McGill University, Canada)

The same concept can be applied in managing maxillofacial defects secondary to large tumors resections. It is extremely common to have patients ask their physicians mainly about the "postoperative scar" rather than the outcome of the tumor resection margin which the treating physician spends a lot of time trying to explain [4]. Although that assuring total tumor resection and free margins can be the surgeons main nightmare in treating such large invasive tumors, restoring facial esthetics is a primary concern that might even change the treatment process accordingly, not to mention the importance of overall health status, safety of treatment, time and cost effectiveness. A thorough discussion of the treatment benefits, alternatives, and risks with the patient himself and the family is essential to construct the best treatment plan and options.

Tumors can occur in young or elderly individuals; each has its individual treatment concept with regard to restoring the quality of life. Younger ambitious individuals dream of full recovery and return to social life, while older individuals think of their family and their post-surgical facial image and how it will affect them and their offspring. Hence, a treatment plan for a 14 year-old girl suffering from invasive mandibular Ewing's sarcoma will not be managed the same way as a mandible pathology in an 89 year-old grandfather. In this chapter, we will discuss some cases with variable facial defects that are treated considering the points mentioned. The cases presented were considered as severe in its category.

In the midst of all the surgical challenges, it is important to realize that achieving the combined goals is not always an easy task. Achieving full function, perfect occlusion and esthetics in a major referral center with a long waiting list of patients can be a busy surgeon's biggest nightmare.

Case 1: Secondary upper lip deformity.

This is a case that discusses a secondary reconstructive operation for a known cleft lip and palate patient who is not satisfied with the results. A 22-year - old female patient treated for cleft lip and palate in various centers across the country. She came to our clinic with a complaint of deformed upper liplocated more posterior than the lower lip. In addition, she did not like how her nose appeared. Clinical exam showed a thin upper lip, inverted, and located posterior to the lower lip. The frontal evaluation showed a thin flat upper lip, undefined white roll, uneven vermilion border, undefined cupids bow and philtrum edges. Further, the lower lip showed more volume and definition. The nose was also deformed and in a very bad condition and displayed poor results of previous rhinoplasty procedures (Figures 2, 3). Several surgeons have met the patient and recommended midface augmentation and possible LeFort 1 osteotomy and advancement inorder to correct the midface deficiency and give her nose some projection and upward rotation. The patient was afraid to go through this procedure and asked me if other treatment options can be offered to her. On clinical and radiographic investigations, its was apparent that the upper lip soft tissue disfigurement comprised a major area of the problem which a Le Fort 1 advancement alone may not be able to correct especially since the patient had an acceptable dental occlusion. Alternatively, the patient was offered the following surgical plan:

1. Upper lip lift and eversion chieloplasty

2. Abdomen fat transfer to the upper lip

3. Delayed reconstructive rhinoplasty and lip border definition

The patient agreed to the surgical plan, and the procedure was accomplished under general anesthesia. The flap design, W-plasty with asymmetric arms to reconstruct the deformed philtrum, philtum edges, cupids bow, and white roll alignment are shown in Figures 4-6. [5]. The patient had a flat asymmetric inverted lip, which made selection of the lifting direction more challenging. The underlying muscle layer was identified and resection of the planned W-skin was made. Minimal flap undermining was done in a caudal direction only and an attempt to evaluate the eversion movement was performed to assess the need of any further excision. After the chieloplasty was accomplished, fat was harvested from the right abdominal area and transferred to the upper lip and vermillion area. Over- correction was performed to compensate for the postoperative fat resorption. Polygalactin 90, 4-0 suture was used to approximate the subcutaneous tissue and nylon 6-0 suture was used to close the skin layer.

The operation went well and the patient was transferred to the ward the day of the operation and was discharged from the hospital in three days. She was prescribed antibiotics, analgesics, and a postoperative instruction sheet that include sun protection advice. The recovery period was uneventful. The postoperative figures showing the lip new look, which was well appreciated by the patient and her family.

Postoperatively the patient was seen and plans were made to pursue the secondary rhinoplasty in 6 months. However, the patient failed to refer for follow up as she got married and moved into another city.

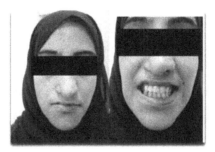

Figure 2. Frontal view showing the severe upper lip inversion, loss of mass, flat archititcure and loss of philtum anatomy cupids bow and tuberculum.

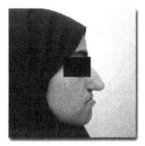

Figure 3. profile image showing the severe upper lip retro positioned, flat, and atrophic mass when compared to the upper lip, simulating a midface dificiency condition.

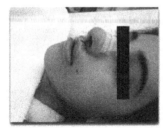

Figure 4. One day postoperatively showing the upper lip improved shape, thickness, and position in relation to the lower lip.

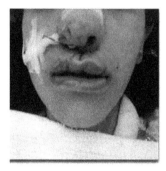

Figure 5. one day postoperatively showing the improved shape and thickness of the upper lip after the fat transfer graft.

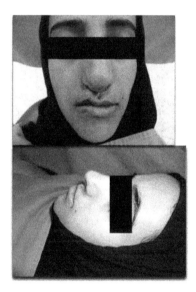

Figure 6. days postoperatively

Case 2: Panfacial fracture.

This case, discusses a scenario where flap design should be planned in order to achieve multiple surgical objectives. Here it was prudent to use the primary laceration line, expose the fracture sites, and to obtain soft tissue lifting where needed. An 18 year-old female patient was a victim of a severe road traffic accident. She was admitted to the hospital for general systemic stabilization. She was cleared for operation about one month post-admission. Clinical examination showed right temporal degloving laceration that was sutured in the emergency department. A drooping right eyebrow, and displaced zygomatic prominence into inferior medial position was apparent. The skin showed multiple abrasions of the right side of the face, periorbital region and cheek, which felt to be fibrosed, and fixed to the underlying tissue.The CT scan showed severely displaced right ZMC fracture into inferior-medial-posterior direction with displaced zygomatic arch fracture (Figures 7, 8). After discussing the case with the patient and her family, the plan was to extend the temporal degloving laceration into a coronal and pre auricular flap in order to expose the fractures and the zygomatic arch. Under general anesthesia, the patient underwent the planned flap design, and all the fracture sites were exposed successfully. Open reduction of the fractures and re-orienting the ZMC back to anterior-lateral-superior direction was accomplished concomitantly via fixating the zygomatic arch and facial fractures using plates and screws. Although fracture reduction and fixation was pursued to achieve symmetry with the contralateral side as much as possible, it was clear to the surgical team that soft tissue closure of a defect of such extent will not help the preoperative facial ptosis [6]. Hence, our approach was to give the right facial aspect some brow and facelift through the opened flap. The procedure was attempted in two planes, a deeper plane to the border of the zygomatic prominence just deep to McGregors patch, using 3-0 polygalactin 90 sutures were used to resuspend the deeper structures in an upward and lateral direction. The second plane was more superficial and excess skin and subcutaneous tissue was trimmed and the face and brow were lifted with minor over correction compared to other side to compensate for postoperative fibrosis. The lifting procedure added approximately 30 minutes to the operating time, as the surgical plan and flap design was used simultaneously for common objectives. Final closure was attempted using 3-0 polygalactin 90 suture for the subcutaneous plane and staples for the skin. An external head ribbon dressing was applied to support the lifting procedure (Figures 9-12). The patient returned to the ICU and stayed in the hospital for 4 more weeks before leaving into a neurological rehabilitation center.

The patient was seen couple of months later and the lifting procedure showed acceptable facial symmetry, although she will require further skin rejuvenation procedures for the skin abrasion wounds.

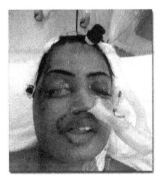

Figure 7. Frontal view of panfacial fracture on day 6 after trauma.

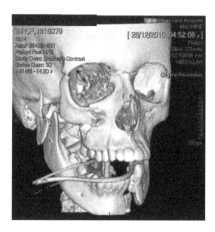

Figure 8. Preoperative 3D CT scan simulation showing the right ZMC complex displaced fracture.

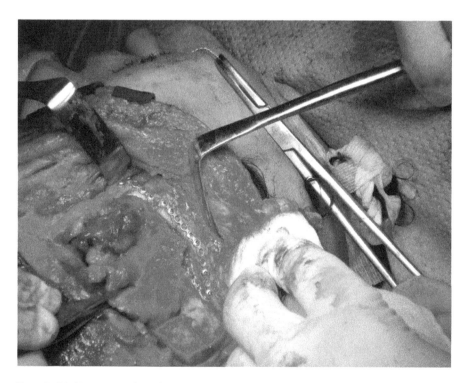

Figure 9. clinical intraoperative figure showing zygomatic arch reduction and fixation.

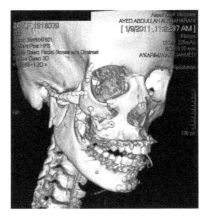

Figure 10. A postoperative 3D CT simulation image showing the perfect fracture reduction and fixation, however, soft management was still needed to optimize the clinical results.

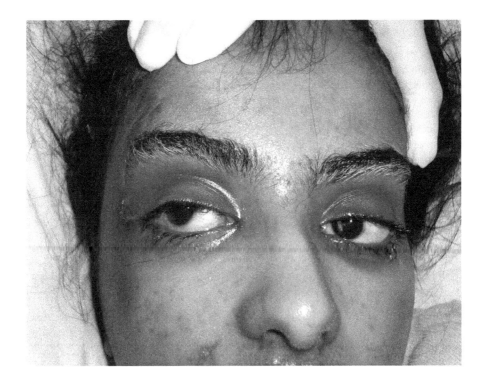

Figure 11. Right eyebrow overcorrection to compensate for future reduction.

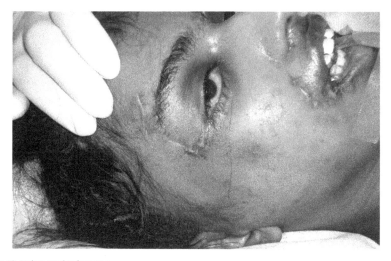

Figure 12. Right periorbital scarring.

Case 3: Atrophic mandible fracture secondary to anterior implant placement.

This case discusses the importance of evaluating the skin type and architecture before attempting a transcervical approach to the mandible. Although the intraoral approach does have the advantages of avoiding scar, avoiding the risk of facial nerve injury, and less emotional impact on patients, it is not inapplicable in all cases. Hence, case selection is the main factor to consider to pursue the approach [7]. A 77 year-old female patient came to our clinic after having five anterior dental implants placed in the mandibular interformanial area. Her chief complaint was pain at the right first premolar implant site. The patient had her implants placed 4 days before sensing a crack while eating using her provisional denture. Her clinical and radiographic investigations showed that she had a compound displaced atrophic mandible fracture at the implant site. The patient had a thin overall body architecture and thin skin – subcutaneous envelope in the head and neck region. The elasticity of the skin showed slow return on snap elasticity test.Usually the treatment of atrophic mandible fracture is through a transcervical incision for sufficient exposure and manipulation. Drawbacks of transcervical approach include risk of injury to the marginal mandibular nerve, unesthetic scar, and risk of transcutaneous fistula in elderly patients. However, considering the body and skin quality of the patient, an intra oral approach was considered to mainly reduce the chances of unesthetic scarring, and transcutaneous fistula.

The procedure was explained to the patient and she expressed total interest in avoiding the transcervical approach. An intraoral approach was performed as anticipated and sufficient access for plate fixation at the symphysis and parasymphysis areas while a transbuccal trocar access was used for plate fixation of the body and angle. The incision was placed at the crest of the mandible with two distal vertical releases to elevate a fullthickness flap. The mental nerves were identified and protected throughout the procedure. Reduction and fixation of the fracture was done using 2.4 locking plate and screws. To prepare for closure, the flap at the lower lip side was undermined to achieve tension free approximation at the anterior segment. The mentalis muscle and flap were then reapproximated using 3-0 polygalactin 90 suture. An external dressing was placed on the chin and used for 2 weeks (Figures 13-18).

Postoperativeradiographs showed adequate plate and screw positioning. The patient was started on clear fluid diet and was discharged from the hospital on the third postoperative day. At the 1.5 year follow up visit showed cosmetic facial results and the patient is satisfied with the results of treatment.

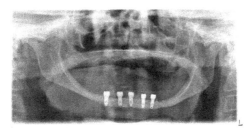

Figure 13. Panormaic radiograph showing the mandible fracture site at the right body region at the right premolar site.

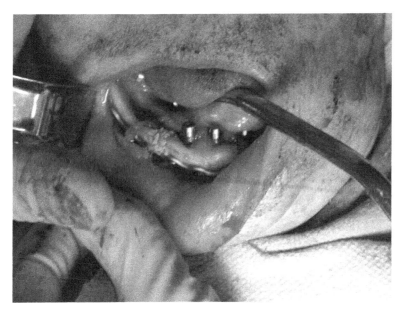

Figure 14. Reconstruction plate is in place and the fracture gap grafted with autogenous bone. Note the integrity of the mental nerve.

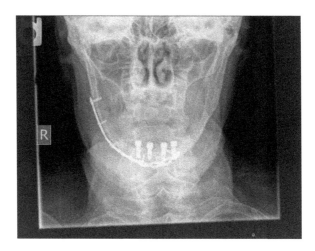

Figure 15. AP radiograph showing the reconstruction plate in place and the challenging screw position in between the implants.

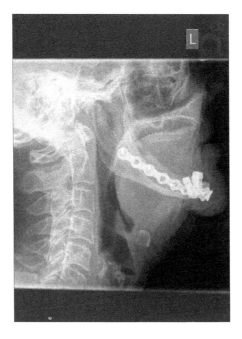

Figure 16. A lateral cephalometric radiograph showing the reconstruction plate in place at the most inferior border of the severely atrophic mandible.

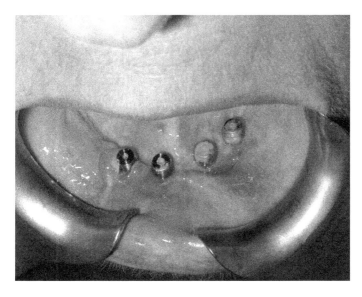

Figure 17. 5 weeks postoperative occlusal picture. Showing good closure of the wound all over including the previously dehisced site on the left implants area.

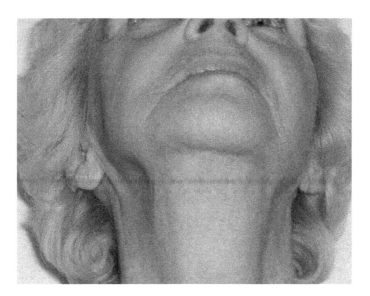

Figure 18. A clinical picutre of the cervical region 3 months postoperatively showing cosmetically acceptable neck area that was not affected by the surgical intevention.

Case 4: Bilateral cleft lip and palate with severe displacement of the premaxilla in a 17 year-old female (Figures 19-24).

This case shows a rare case of severe facial disfigurement secondary to neglected cleft lip and palate (CLAP) management from birth to the age of 17. This 17 year- old female patient referred to our clinic complaining of her facial deformity that negatively affected her social life and education to such an extent that she had to stop going to school. On clinical and ra-diographic examination, the patient had bilateral CLAP with severe (3.7cm) premaxillary displacement in an anterior and inferior position. She reported she had not sought professio-nal medical help during the past 17 years of her life [8]. As the facial reconstruction team had to deal with a severe CLAP facial disfigurement in an older patient, the surgical plan mainly focused on accelerating the possibility of having this girl reintegrating back into so-cial life and continuing education. Hence, it was planned to surgically reposition the pre-maxilla and repair the cleft palatal severe defect concomitantly.

The patient was informed that further reconstructive surgeries such as revision chieloplasty, rhinoplasty, oral rehabilitation, and possibly orthognathic surgeries might be required in the future.

Under general anesthesia, the patient's wide cleft palate was identified and planned for clo-sure of the uvula, soft and hard palate defect using full thickness total palatal flaps (V-Y pushback) and vomerian flaps concomitantly with premaxilla reduction and nasal septum flap management.The wide cleft palate was managed successfully and the protruded pre-maxilla/septum bone was resected (2.9cm) in semi triangular shape to help in repositioning the premaxilla in back-upward direction. The nasal septum had to be trimmed conservative-ly and the premax position was secured using 4-0 Prolene sutures fixated at the bony seg-ments of the palate and premaxilla. Minimal gengivo-periosteoplasty adhesion was made at the proximal segment to aid in retaining the new position in tension free fashion.

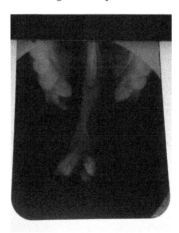

Figure 19. An occlusal view showing the severe premaxilla displacement.

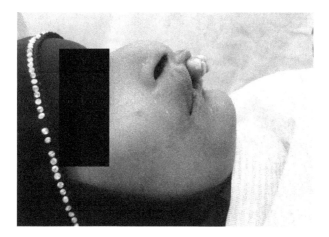

Figure 20. Lateral Profile view.

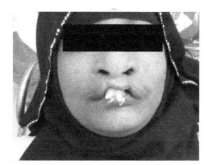

Figure 21. Frontal view.

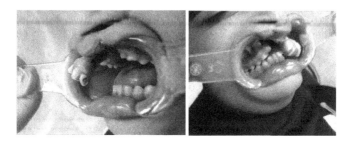

Figure 22. Lateral occlusal view.

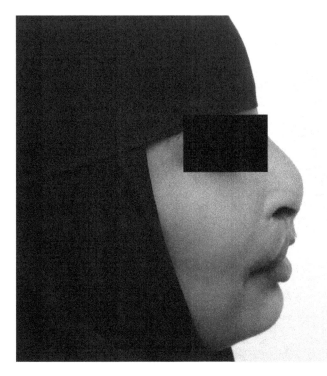

Figure 23. One week postoperative profile picture showing that the premaxilla is now enclosed back inside the oral cavity after resecting about 2.9cm of the protruded premaxillary bone and nasal septum reduction.

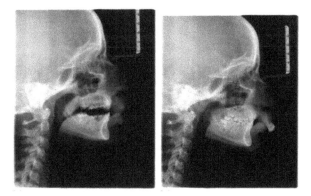

Figure 24. Lateral cephalometric showing the difference between the preoperative position (right) and on the post-operative reduced position (Left).

Case 5: Severe orbital vertical dystopia.

A 20 year- old male patient referred complaining of severe unesthetic vertical dystopia. The patient had a history of RTA few months ago and was in the ICU to control his unstable systemic status. Maxillofacial surgeries were not attempted for him at that time. Clinical examination revealed right orbital vertical dystopia of about 2cm inferiorly, fibrotic skin abrasions at the nasoorbital ethmoidal region, at the cheek, forehead, and lateral orbital regions. Due to the aforementioned, the patient was off school for one year since the patient planed to pursue facial reconstruction before enrolling back to school. Radiographic interpretation revealed orbital floor fracture and inferior displacement into the maxillary sinus by 2cm. ENT consultation was done and interpreted normal functioning status of the maxillary sinus. Management of such cases is challenging since the deformity is secondary to untreated displaced facial fractures a year ago and all the fractures have healed in abnormal alignment pattern. Furthermore, the soft tissue was deformed due to malunion and poor skin texture due to the scarring. The surgical objective was to alleviate the unesthetic vertical dystopia using a block of nonvascularized bone from the anterior iliac crest to support the eyeball superiorly, realign the inferior orbital rim which was posteriorly displaced, lift the right brow upwards and laterally, and canthoplasty for the deformed lateral canthus. Under general anesthesia, a transconjuctival incision with lateral canthotomy was performed to expose the inferior orbital rim and displaced orbital floor [9]. Elevation of the eyeball was attempted and the space of the supporting block was prepared. A second team was harvesting the anterior iliac crest bone graft, which was trimmed and sandwiched under the eyeball with consideration to reconstruct the inferior orbital rim and anteroposterior defect. Next, canthopexy of the lateral canthal tendons was done in a more superior position to compensate for the traumatic inferior displacement. The brow was lifted using the scar revision incision at the superior orbital rim area. (Figures 25-29) Follow up visits were uneventful and showed significant improvement and patient satisfaction. The patient is still planned for further reconstructive surgeries and skin rejuvenation procedures and he is already enrolled back to school.

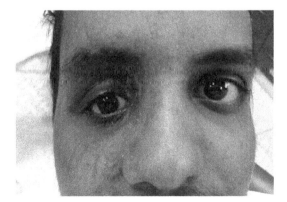

Figure 25. Right orbital inferior vertical dystopia.

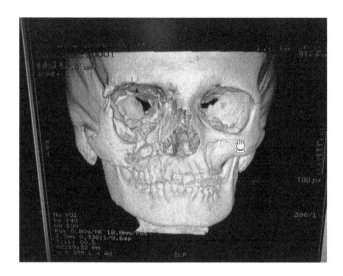

Figure 26. CT 3d simulation showing the magnitude of the inferior right dystopia.

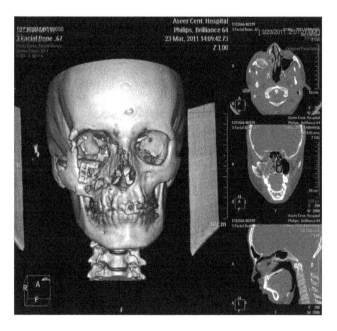

Figure 27. Postoperative 3D CT simulation showing the magnitude of right inferior orbital rim and floor elevation using a non vascularized bone graft from the anterior iliac crest.

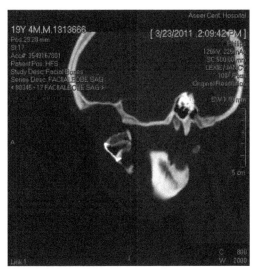

Figure 28. a postoperative CT scan of parasagittal cut showing section of the graft material that is elevating the eye ball back into the orbital cavity.

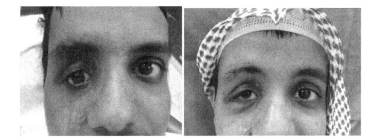

Figure 29. The left view is the preoperative view showing the vertical dystopia while the right showing the postoperative correction of the dystopia and brow lift, as the first stage of treatment. Further corrective surgeries are planned.

2. Conclusion

This chapter presents five cases with facial deformities that are considered "severe". All five cases share the fact that facial esthetics was a significant consideration in the plan of management. Planning the flap design, hard tissue management, and soft tissue management are the basic pillars of treatment. As each of the three pillars of facial reconstruction contribute to the surgical procedure, equal attention should be paid to each. The aim of this chapter was to high-light the importance of this issue in treating oral maxillofacial patients.

Acknowledgements

The author would like to thank Dr. Morai Alqahtani and Dr Bader A. Raouf (Plastic Surgery Department, Saudi Arabia) for their assistance and support towards the Maxillofacial Surgery and Reconstruction Department, Dr Tord Lundgren (Periodontics surgery – USA, Sweden / Saudi Arabia) and Dr Ibrahim Zabani (Anesthesia – Saudi Arabia) for their help in solving the obstacles for treating the facial deformity patients, Dr Joe III Nimatu (Richmond, Virginia, USA) for his continuous insights in the field of facial cosmetics, my deep gratitude to the higher management of Umm Al Qura University – College of Dentistry for the strong support to the field of research, and last but not least "my family; Najiah, Ghena, and Ibrahim" in the beautiful Jeddah city of Saudi Arabia for their patience and support throughout all the working hours outside as well as inside home, thank you all.

Author details

Mazen Almasri

Address all correspondence to: mazen_ajm@yahoo.com

Assistant Professor of Oral Maxillofacial Surgery and Reconstruction Faculty of Dentistry, Umm Alqura University, Saudi Arabia

References

[1] Aksoy, E., Unlü, E., & Sensöz, O. (2002). A retrospective study on epidemiology and treatment of maxillofacial fractures. *J Craniofac surg.*, 13(6), 772-5.

[2] Miloro, Michael. (2004). Peterson's Principle's of Oral and Maxillofacial Surgery. *BC DECKER INC.*, 327.

[3] Ozkaya, O., Turgut, G., Kayali, M. U., Uğurlu, K., Kuran, I., & Baş, L. (2009). A retrospective study on the epidemiology and treatment of maxillofacial fractures. *Ulus Travma Acil Cerrahi Derg.*, 15(3), 262-6.

[4] Binahmed, A., Nason, R. W., & Abdoh, A. A. (2007). The clinical significance of the positive surgical margin in oral cancer. *Oral Oncol.*, 43(8), 780-4.

[5] Waldman, S. R. (2007). The subnasal lift. *Facial Plast Surg Clin North Am.*, 15(4), 513-6.

[6] Ranganath, K., & Hemanth Kumar, H. R. (2011). The correction of post-traumatic pan facial residual deformity. *J Maxillofac Oral Surg.*, 10(1), 20-4.

[7] Almasri, M., & El -Hakim, M. (2012). Fracture of the anterior segment of the atrophic mandible related to dental implants. *Int J Oral Maxillofac Surg.*, 41(5), 646-9, Epub 2012 Feb 5.

[8] Dürwald, J., & Dannhauer, K. H. (2007). Vertical development of the cleft segments in infants with bilateral cleft lip and palate: effect of dentofacial orthopedic and surgical treatment on maxillary morphology from birth to the age of 11 months. *J Orofac Orthop.*, 68(3), 183-97.

[9] Moore, F. O., Thornton, B. P., Zabel, D. D., & Vasconez, H. C. (2004). Autogenous orbital reconstruction in a child with congenital abnormalities of the orbital roof and vertical orbital dystopia. *J Craniofac Surg.*, 15(6), 930-3.

Permissions

The contributors of this book come from diverse backgrounds, making this book a truly international effort. This book will bring forth new frontiers with its revolutionizing research information and detailed analysis of the nascent developments around the world.

We would like to thank Mohammad Hosein Kalantar Motamedi, DDS, for lending his expertise to make the book truly unique. He has played a crucial role in the development of this book. Without his invaluable contribution this book wouldn't have been possible. He has made vital efforts to compile up to date information on the varied aspects of this subject to make this book a valuable addition to the collection of many professionals and students.

This book was conceptualized with the vision of imparting up-to-date information and advanced data in this field. To ensure the same, a matchless editorial board was set up. Every individual on the board went through rigorous rounds of assessment to prove their worth. After which they invested a large part of their time researching and compiling the most relevant data for our readers. Conferences and sessions were held from time to time between the editorial board and the contributing authors to present the data in the most comprehensible form. The editorial team has worked tirelessly to provide valuable and valid information to help people across the globe.

Every chapter published in this book has been scrutinized by our experts. Their significance has been extensively debated. The topics covered herein carry significant findings which will fuel the growth of the discipline. They may even be implemented as practical applications or may be referred to as a beginning point for another development. Chapters in this book were first published by InTech; hereby published with permission under the Creative Commons Attribution License or equivalent.

The editorial board has been involved in producing this book since its inception. They have spent rigorous hours researching and exploring the diverse topics which have resulted in the successful publishing of this book. They have passed on their knowledge of decades through this book. To expedite this challenging task, the publisher supported the team at every step. A small team of assistant editors was also appointed to further simplify the editing procedure and attain best results for the readers.

Our editorial team has been hand-picked from every corner of the world. Their multi-ethnicity adds dynamic inputs to the discussions which result in innovative outcomes. These outcomes are then further discussed with the researchers and contributors who give their valuable feedback and opinion regarding the same. The feedback is then collaborated with the researches and they are edited in a comprehensive manner to aid the understanding of the subject.

Apart from the editorial board, the designing team has also invested a significant amount of their time in understanding the subject and creating the most relevant covers. They scrutinized every image to scout for the most suitable representation of the subject and create an appropriate cover for the book.

The publishing team has been involved in this book since its early stages. They were actively engaged in every process, be it collecting the data, connecting with the contributors or procuring relevant information. The team has been an ardent support to the editorial, designing and production team. Their endless efforts to recruit the best for this project, has resulted in the accomplishment of this book. They are a veteran in the field of academics and their pool of knowledge is as vast as their experience in printing. Their expertise and guidance has proved useful at every step. Their uncompromising quality standards have made this book an exceptional effort. Their encouragement from time to time has been an inspiration for everyone.

The publisher and the editorial board hope that this book will prove to be a valuable piece of knowledge for researchers, students, practitioners and scholars across the globe.

List of Contributors

Sertac Aktop, Onur Gonul, Tulin Satilmis, Hasan Garip and Kamil Goker
Department of Oral and Maxillofacial Surgery, Marmara University, Istanbul, Turkey

Amrish Bhagol, Virendra Singh
Department of Oral and Maxillofacial Surgery, Post Graduate Institute of Dental Sciences, Pt. B.D. Sharma University of Health Sciences, Rohtak, Haryana, India

Ruchi Singhal
Department of Pedodontic and Preventive Dentistry, Post Graduate Institute of Dental Sciences, Pt. B.D. Sharma University of Health Sciences, Rohtak, Haryana, India

Hossein Behnia
Department of Oral and Maxillofacial Surgery, School of Dentistry, Shahid Beheshti University of Medical Sciences, Tehran, Iran

Azita Tehranchi
Department of Orthodontics, School of Dentistry, Shahid Beheshti University of Medical Sciences, Tehran, Iran

Golnaz Morad
Dental Research Center, Shahid Beheshti University of Medical Sciences, Tehran, Iran

Shahram Nazerani
Associate Professor of Surgery, Firouzgar Hospital, Teheran, Iran
Tehran University of Medical Sciences, Tehran, Iran

Maiolino Thomaz Fonseca Oliveira, Flaviana Soares Rocha, Jonas Dantas Batista and Darceny Zanetta-Barbosa
Department of Oral and Maxillofacial Surgery and Implantology – School of Dentistry - Federal University of Uberlândia – UFU, Brazil

Sylvio Luiz Costa de Moraes
Head, Clinic for Cranio-Maxillofacial Surgery at Hospital São Francisco, Director of Facial Reconstruction Center – RECONFACE, Faculty AO-Foundation

Mohammad Hosein Kalantar Motamedi
Professor of Oral and Maxillofacial Surgery, Trauma Research Center, Baqiyatallah University of Medical Sciences, and Attending Surgeon, Azad University of Medical Sciences, Tehran, Iran

Seyed Hossein Mortazavi, Hossein Behnia and Masoud Yaghmaei
Professor of Oral and Maxillofacial Surgery, Department of Oral and Maxillofacial Surgery, Taleghani Medical Center, Shahid Beheshti University of Medical Sciences, Tehran, Iran

Abbas Khodayari, Fahimeh Akhlaghi, Mohammad Ghasem Shams
Associate Professor of Oral and Maxillofacial Surgery, Department of Oral and Maxillofacial Surgery, Taleghani Medical Center, Shahid Beheshti University of Medical Sciences, Tehran, Iran

Rashid Zargar Marandi
Neurosurgeon, Department of Neurosurgery, Baqiyatallah University of Medical Sciences, Tehran, Iran

Koroush Taheri Talesh
Oral and Maxillofacial Surgery Tabriz University of Medical Sciences and Azad University of Medical Sciences, Tehran, Iran

Mohammad Hosein Kalantar Motamedi
Oral and Maxillofacial Surgery Baqiyatallah University of Medical Sciences Trauma Research Center, Tehran, Iran

Tarek El-Bialy
Faculty of Medicine and Dentistry, 7-020D Katz Group Centre for Pharmacy and Health Research, University of Alberta, Edmonton, Alberta, Canada

Adel Alhadlaq
College of Dentistry, King Saud University, Riyadh, Saudi Arabia

Mazen Almasri
Assistant Professor of Oral Maxillofacial Surgery and Reconstruction Faculty of Dentistry, Umm Alqura University, Saudi Arabia